'This book celebrates all that yoga is. I[?] and shows us that yoga has open arms practise. A liberating look at how anyor[?] has to offer mentally and physically. Do[?] past experiences to show us the origins and how we can all be more inclusive ... celebration of yoga for all.'

– Fearne Cotton

'As a yoga teacher and teacher trainer, I'm always in search of resources for aspiring teachers (and for myself!) that are practical, helpful and, most importantly, represent my values. Donna Noble's new book *Teaching Body Positive Yoga* meets all of these criteria and then some. I highly recommend it to all yoga teachers and future teachers. Even if you think you "don't need this book", you need this book.'

– Kat (Heagberg) Rebar, co-author of Yoga Where You Are *and former Editor-in-Chief* Yoga International

'In *Teaching Body Positive Yoga*, Donna Noble has written a superbly relatable, practical book. She gives us the why as well as the how to practise inclusive, Body Positive Yoga. I especially love the section called Body Positive Yoga Off the Mat where Noble gives us case studies and practices to bring these tools into every moment of our lives! She confidently states, "As teachers you have a voice that is able to create yoga's future." She gives us many tools and practices to create a more inclusive future. As a South Asian woman working to preserve the heart of yoga today, I'm thrilled to have Noble's book grace my yoga bookshelves and support all of our practice and teaching.'

– Susanna Barkataki, author of Embrace Yoga's Roots

'Donna distills the most fundamental information about diversity and inclusivity in yoga, making it a must-read for anyone in the industry.'

– Reeva Misra, Founder and CEO of Walking on Earth

'Donna Noble is a tireless, fearless, inspirational and fierce campaigner for anyone who feels that they have become invisible in the world of westernised wellness with a simple message for everyone and everybody, reflected in every single page of this marvellous book: you are welcome on the yoga mat. This book, and Donna's knowledge and commitment, represents a vital contribution not only toward body positive yoga, but toward dismantling the many cultural issues and obstacles that stand in the way of this practice being accessible to all.'

– *Dr Lee Watson, Founder of Fierce Calm*

'Donna Noble writes in a way that allows the reader to understand the universality of yoga as a beautiful ancient practice. Stripping away all the notions that make yoga as we know it in the West to feel inaccessible, Donna reminds us that to be in the present is to be at one with the body mind and soul. Amazing work!'

– *Kelechi Okafor, actress and Co-founder*
of Kelechnekoff Fitness Studio

'If you're looking to better understand and inform yourself with topics like the history of body positivity, and the use and understanding of language on and off the yoga mat, then this is a great guide for you; well-researched and easy to digest.'

– *Lindsey Porter, yogi, yoga tutor and author of*
Whirlpools, Yoga and The Balance of Life

'It was such a pleasure reading *Teaching Body Positive Yoga*! Thank you for creating this important resource! The case studies at the end of the book were extremely moving as well as maddening. It is a reminder that so much work still needs to be done to make sure yoga is inclusive for all body types, ethnicities, ages, genders or abilities. *Teaching Body Positive Yoga* should be required reading in all teacher training courses.'

– *Lauren Cap, writer*

'Donna Noble's *Teaching Body Positive Yoga* is a jewel in my yoga library. It acknowledges that we live in bodies of various sizes, races, genders and mobilities – and that we bring different embodied experiences to the mat. Her approach to yoga respects whatever body we are practising in. She offers wisdom from years of practice, solid research and personal experience – so her guidance feels trustworthy and honourable.'

– Tamara Jeffries, Senior Editor of Yoga Journal

'Donna's book not only encourages the reader to think about the necessity of making the yoga industry affirming and accessible for all bodies, but she gives them the tools and skills to put what they're reading into practice in actionable and meaningful ways. Everyone in the yoga industry needs to read this book.'

– Chrissy King, writer, speaker, Fitness and Strength Coach and Creator of The Body Liberation Project™

'Donna Noble has crafted a deeply uplifting, accessible and thought-provoking text imploring the reader to consider boundaries to yoga practice and how to mindfully dissemble them in practical and systematic ways. As she poignantly notes, "Every Body is a Yoga Body". For this adage to manifest we must all look at and beyond our preconceived ideas. Through first-person accounts and life experience, Noble shares the truly yogic pursuit of divesting oneself of staunchly held biases allowing us to expand our vision of what yoga and yoga practitioners look like. In reading her book, it is clear that Body Positivity Yoga is and should be the future of yoga.'

– Heather Mason, Founder of Minded Institute

Teaching Body Positive Yoga

of related interest

Yoga Teaching Handbook
A Practical Guide for Yoga Teachers and Trainees
Edited by Sian O'Neill
ISBN 978 1 84819 355 0
eISBN 978 0 85701 313 2

Chair Yoga
Seated Exercises for Health and Wellbeing
Edeltraud Rohnfeld
Illustrated by Edeltraud Rohnfeld
ISBN 978 1 84819 078 8
eISBN 978 0 85701 056 8

Theming Skills for Yoga Teachers
Tools to Inspire Creative and Connected Classes
Tanja Mickwitz
ISBN 978 1 78775 687 8
eISBN 978 1 78775 688 5
Yoga Teaching Guides

Supporting Yoga Students with Common Injuries and Conditions
A Handbook for Teachers and Trainees
Dr Andrew McGonigle
ISBN 978 1 78775 469 0
eISBN 978 1 78775 470 6
Yoga Teaching Guides

The Yoga Teacher Mentor
A Reflective Guide to Holding Spaces, Maintaining Boundaries, and Creating Inclusive Classes
Jess Glenny
Foreword by Norman Blair
ISBN 978 1 78775 126 2
eISBN 978 1 78775 127 9

TEACHING BODY POSITIVE YOGA

A Guide to Inclusivity, Language and Props

DONNA NOBLE

Foreword by Jivana Heyman

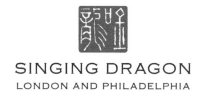

SINGING DRAGON
LONDON AND PHILADELPHIA

First published in Great Britain in 2022 by Singing Dragon,
an imprint of Jessica Kingsley Publishers
An imprint of Hodder & Stoughton Ltd
An Hachette UK Company

3

A CIP catalogue record for this title is available from the
British Library and the Library of Congress

ISBN 978 1 78775 335 8
eISBN 978 1 78775 336 5

Printed and bound by CPI Group (UK) Ltd, Croydon, CR0 4YY

Jessica Kingsley Publishers' policy is to use papers that are natural,
renewable and recyclable products and made from wood grown in
sustainable forests. The logging and manufacturing processes are expected
to conform to the environmental regulations of the country of origin.

Jessica Kingsley Publishers
Carmelite House
50 Victoria Embankment
London EC4Y 0DZ

www.singingdragon.com

This book is dedicated to my late grandmother, Lucille Morgan. May you know that you will always have a place in my heart. Until we meet again...

It is also dedicated to my mother, Emily Phillips, and my grandfather, Vincent Morgan.

Contents

Part 3: Body Positivity off the Yoga Mat

Foreword

Yoga's timeless message is that we're all equal in spirit, and that what we're seeking is found within us. Yet, over the past few decades, yoga has been taught in a way that is exclusive and inaccessible. It's finally time to bring this into alignment: the way we teach and share yoga needs to reflect the teachings themselves. We need to look beyond the superficial messages of contemporary culture to reveal deeper essential truths about yoga and about ourselves.

The history of yoga spans literally thousands of years, and amazingly, the essential philosophy hasn't changed during all that time, because it contains universal spiritual truths. What has changed over aeons is the way yoga is interpreted and practised, and that's now changing again. In the last few years, we've seen a huge shift towards greater cultural awareness within yoga spaces, and a renewed effort to make yoga accessible and equitable to anyone who is interested in this transformative practice.

This shift includes greater respect for the indigenous tradition of yoga, and includes the increased sensitivity of yoga teachers regarding cultural issues such as racism, homophobia, ageism, ableism and fat phobia. We are finally seeing the ways these issues have been obstacles to a practice that is accessible at its heart. There is a generation of yoga teachers who are at the forefront of the shift, such as Dianne Bondy, Matthew Sanford, Amber Karnes, Susanna Barkataki and Jessamyn Stanley – and now we can add Donna Noble to that list.

I can just see Donna's face as she reads that sentence! She will laugh it off, but her humility is her hidden strength. Behind that humble exterior hides a powerful mind that is finally available to the world through this book. I am so excited, and in a way relieved, to see this book being published – not only because it's great to see Donna recognised as a leader in the field, but also because there's so much wisdom here that needs to be shared with the entire yoga community.

Donna has broken down in detail most of the major issues that we need to be talking about in yoga today. The question this book answers is 'How do we share these teachings with everyone?' This is a question I feel equally passionate about answering. I've spent the last 30 years trying to make yoga accessible through my teacher trainings, books and the non-profit I founded, the Accessible Yoga Association.

In fact, I met Donna many years ago when she attended my Accessible Yoga training in London, and I knew the minute I met her that she had a special balance of wisdom and clarity about her that would make her a force to be reckoned with. When I next returned to London, I asked her to assist me in the training. It was wonderful to see her in the role of training teachers, and watch the way they responded to her kindness and experience. Now, we all get to benefit from her wisdom.

What's particularly interesting in this book is the way that Donna integrates a contemporary understanding of body image and diet culture and the many ways they contribute to making yoga inaccessible. Modern yoga has a major image problem, and that's what Donna has so brilliantly dismantled here, one misunderstanding at a time. It's like she has taken down a wall brick by brick so that we can access the heart of the teachings – no longer hidden and out of reach.

As Donna explains, 'True body positivity is when everyone is welcome on the yoga mat. You can do this by creating a space where people feel empowered to let their practice accommodate their body and do yoga in a way that feels good for them, so they have agency over their body.' I couldn't agree more. I hope that everyone feels welcome on the yoga mat (or chair), and that they can practise in a way that connects them to their internal power. I also hope that all yoga teachers and practitioners get to read this book, and reflect on the ways that these ancient teachings can be shared in a more sensitive and beneficial way.

Jivana Heyman

Acknowledgements

There are so many people who I need to thank. The list is endless.

I am so grateful to my family for always believing in and supporting me even when they have not always understood my journey. Me being happy was enough for them.

To my dear friend Lindsey Porter, who has provided invaluable support. The idea for the book came from her, when without hesitation she facilitated the introduction to my publishers.

To everyone who was part of my journey. These people inspired and supported me during what was a new and unknown process, even when I had doubts about ever finishing this book. I am so grateful for their belief in me, especially those I bored talking endlessly about the process.

Deborah Coughlin, for writing the article in *The Guardian* that started it all, giving me the courage to start my body positive journey.

I am grateful to the teachers who shared their knowledge and experience during my yoga journey. Dianne Bondy and Amber Karnes, my first body positive yoga teachers, for showing me how to create safe spaces for those invisible within the yoga community. Jessamyn Stanley, for inspiring me and for donating her time at my first Body Positive workshop. Jivana Heyman, for sharing his infinite wisdom on how to teach mixed-level classes and writing the amazing foreword.

Special thanks to Twanna Doherty and Yogamatters for their amazing photography and support. Also for letting me see the importance of being on the cover. Big thanks to the main models, Affy Uffort, Saskia Bolscher and Mirella Scarborough.

I would like to take this opportunity to show my gratitude to all the contributors who were honest with their opinions and experiences. Detailed information can be found about them at the end of the book.

I would like to thank everyone who donated to the crowdfunding campaign to have my first stand at Om Yoga Show. This was going to allow me to see if there really was a need for something like Curvesomeyoga, to show that every body is a yoga body.

To those who are invisible and are not convinced that yoga or wellbeing is their birthright. I hope that sharing what I have learnt during my yoga journey will help to go some way to helping those who are afraid to get on the yoga mat.

I would also like to acknowledge the incredible patience and support of my editor, Sarah Hamlin, and the team at Singing Dragon. They allowed me to find my own way and made my publishing experience so pleasurable.

Finally, a huge thank you to all the students who have trusted me and believed me when I told them that every body is a yoga body! For their patience, which allowed me to grow and develop as a teacher and taught me how to be open and honest.

To everyone who had my back every step of the way!

Big love to you all!

Preface

Body positive yoga is the gift of making yoga available for every-BODY, regardless of age, size, ethnicity, ability or gender.

It is still hard for me to comprehend that I have written this book; being an author was never part of my plan. I am so grateful that I get to experience life in a way that unfolds organically and often surprises me and shows me that going with the flow serves me best.

Teaching Body Positive Yoga was written with the support and patience of family and friends. It is a book that shares the experiences and knowledge that I have acquired since 2012 when I looked around the yoga spaces I occupied and noticed that certain groups of our society were missing. I was spurred into action to see how I could help change this narrative. Although I did not have a clue of the how, I did not allow that to stop me. Doing this work has allowed me to discover my passion and purpose to disrupt and bring about change.

Curvesomeyoga was created in 2015. Thank you Nicola Bird for seeing that my innate wisdom was allowing Curvesomeyoga to unfold even when I was not aware. You kept bringing me back to it even when I wanted to move onto the next shiny thing. You kept me looking in that direction.

I hope that this book will provide you, the yoga teacher, with the confidence and knowledge to be able to help make your yoga classes available to everyone who wishes to practise yoga and does not believe having access to yoga and wellbeing is their birthright or is indeed for them.

I have realised that there are many facets to me – a lot of which have not yet been discovered. I don't like labels, I find them constricting – I like to just be and let my actions and the work I do speak for themselves. I like to fly by the seat of my pants and see what I will be doing next. One thing I know is that being of service and creating change appears to be my path – I am not sure how these will develop but I have a deep sense of knowing and I am okay with that.

Part I

OVERVIEW

Introduction

My yoga journey began in the late 1990s when a colleague saw an image of Madonna with one leg behind her head in Eka Pada Sirasana (one leg behind the head pose). Much to my surprise, she suggested that we give yoga a try and the rest, as they say, is history. My first class was taught by a trainee yoga teacher who kindly offered free yoga classes, so we became her guinea pigs.

At the time, I didn't realise that yoga would play such a significant part in my life and eventually allow me to transition from the corporate to the yoga world. My journey wasn't always a linear one. Yoga would always be the casualty in my efforts to climb the corporate ladder, taking a back seat as I completed my Master's degree and began to work longer hours and take on more responsibilities after being promoted.

It was only after becoming ill with Bell's palsy, causing the right side of my face to become paralysed, and then being made redundant, that I felt able to leave behind the stressful corporate world after approximately 20 years. I'd never predicted this. I'd achieved all the things society had told me were signs of success – the job, the house, the car, and so on – but I came to realise that material possessions do not equate to happiness. I found myself asking, 'What is life all about?' 'Is this all there is to life?' Upon reflection, I was in a state of shock after waking up to discover that my face had become unrecognisable, quite literally overnight.

BELL'S PALSY

Bell's palsy, also known as idiopathic facial palsy, is a form of temporary or permanent facial paralysis or weakness on one side of the face. It results from dysfunction of cranial nerve VII (facial nerve), which directs the muscles on one side of the face, including those that control eye blinking and closing and facial expressions such as smiling. (There are 12 pairs of cranial nerves, identified by Roman numerals.) The facial nerve also carries nerve impulses to the tear glands, the saliva glands and the muscles of a small bone in the middle of the ear. It also transmits taste sensations from the tongue.

For more information, see National Institute of Neurological Disorders and Stroke (2019).

I went from being a very confident person to someone who avoided cameras and hid my face because my smile had become lopsided. The first few times I went out in public, I avoided all eye contact so that I wouldn't have to endure the looks of pity or shock. I unconsciously downplayed the severity of the trauma to friends, which became apparent when I witnessed their shocked reactions when they saw my face for the first time.

Around this time, a good friend, Errol Osborne, suggested that I should have a plan B for my career, something I wasn't initially able to fully comprehend – I was supposedly living the dream in terms of all the things society states that you should work to achieve! But after thinking it through, I decided to do a yoga teacher training course with the idea that it was something I could possibly do after my retirement if ever I became bored.

However, the universe delivered! I was to retire from the corporate world and become a yoga teacher much sooner than I could have anticipated or imagined. The realisation that I was destined for another path became apparent while studying on a neuro-linguistic programming (NLP) Master Practitioner course while I was still in my corporate job.

NEURO-LINGUISTIC PROGRAMMING

NLP was created by Richard Bandler and John Grinder in the US in the 1970s.

> A literal translation of the phrase 'Neuro Linguistic Programming' is that NLP empowers, enables and teaches us to better understand the way our brain (neuro) processes the words we use (linguistic) and how that can impact on our past, present and future (programming). It gives us strategies for observing human behaviour and learning from the best (and worst) of that!
>
> Simply put, change is possible – all you need is a desire to change and a willingness to learn new ways of being...with yourself, your thoughts and with others.
>
> NLP has been defined as the 'users manual for your mind' because studying NLP gives us insights into how our thinking patterns can affect every aspect of our lives. (ANLP International CIC, n.d.)

During the course I was asked what was going on in my life. I explained that I didn't know what to do in terms of my career as my role no longer existed and there was a threat of redundancy. I was told that unconsciously I already knew – when I talked about yoga, I 'lit up', but when I spoke about the corporate life, the opposite happened. In that instant, I decided that as soon as I completed the Triyoga teacher training course, I would fly to Los Angeles at the earliest opportunity to attend the hot yoga teacher training. At that stage all I wanted to do was to become a hippy, carefree yoga teacher with no responsibilities, who would just rock up to class and teach and then chill once I was done. This is what being a yoga teacher looked like to me – little did I know what I was letting myself in for in my new career path!

What was meant to be only a nine-week training in the US morphed into six months of travelling. Teaching first in New York and subsequently in Texas, my trip became an unofficial sabbatical. My friends say that once I got on that plane, I was no longer the same person. I started to embrace the 'go with the flow' ethos, and once I began to have faith and trust the process I received daily examples affirming that I was on the right path. Years later, it is still my philosophy.

How did I become a body positive advocate?

I didn't intentionally set out to become a body positive advocate. All I wanted was to share how yoga helped me to heal from the trauma of Bell's palsy, both mentally (in addressing the aspects of my life that were not making me happy) and physically (during the five years it took for my face to begin to recover from the paralysis). I wanted to show how amazing the body is; the more I embraced a yogic path, the more it allowed me to heal. It might sound like a cliché, but it's true: yoga changed my life. It opened me up to opportunities that I could never have imagined and became my vehicle for change and transformation.

Another key turning point in my journey was reading an article in *The Guardian* by Deborah Coughlin titled 'Fat girls do yoga too' (2014), about her dispiriting experience as a yogi. The article led me down a path where I discovered yoga teachers and students like Dianne Bondy, Jessamyn Stanley and Dana Falsetti, and so many more, who shared their practice and demonstrated that yoga was for everyone. I have since had the pleasure of meeting these and many other inspirational yogis. Coughlin's article had a profound effect on me and I couldn't stop talking about it. It came to the point where my friends were palpably bored by my new-found enthusiasm and told me that I needed to either 'shut up or do something about it'. So I took their advice, and later that year created Curvesomeyoga to help make yoga more inclusive and diverse.

My initial aim was to address the issues highlighted by Deborah Coughlin in her article and create a community for individuals who didn't think that yoga was for them because they didn't have what the mainstream yoga industry portrays as a 'yoga body'. Upon reflection, I also wanted to atone for the teachers and students who weren't very welcoming to Deborah and make sure that no one else had the same horrible experience that she did. Here are some words from Deborah about the reaction to the article:

> That article went viral. I was suddenly getting messages from around the globe. Weight Watchers offered me a column. I was offered free yoga stuff. I had clearly hit a nerve. Back in 2014, when I wrote it, yoga was literally marketed as if only skinny, white, blonde women did it – I think a lot has changed since then.
>
> There was already a movement in North America with Dianne Bondy spearheading Black women and bigger women in yoga. But there was nothing like that here in the UK. For whatever reason, we had accepted that yoga was for people who looked like they were living some *Sex in the City* dream.
>
> The fourth wave of feminism has helped change that. Activist and academic language seeped into the mainstream, giving us all the lexicon to challenge the status quo. The rise of Instagram allowed all types of women to put their bodies centre stage and advertising has been forced to follow.
>
> It would still be perfectly reasonable for any woman to feel anxious going into a yoga class or gym or SUP [stand-up paddleboard] lesson. There's a lot of shame, and deeply ingrained fat phobia and racism, that won't go away just because Special K® have made their adverts a bit more inclusive. And so every time I see a woman overcome those massive cultural pressures, to feel the joy of playing in their body, I am moved. (Deborah Coughlin, writer and founder of a mental health tech company; personal communication)

There was clearly a need, a gap in the market, to make yoga more welcoming for those in larger, or non-mainstream-conforming bodies. Just like Deborah, I believed the tide had started to turn, as we slowly began to see a very different image, which was challenging what had become the norm. It was refreshing and exciting to see yogis who looked like me and those who were invisible in yoga. As Deborah said, a lot has already changed since then, but more needs to be done to make all people in all bodies feel accepted in yoga classes.

The mission statement of Curvesomeyoga is very simply 'to show that every body is a yoga BODY!'

First, I needed a name. I wanted something easily recognisable and non-triggering that would appeal to anyone wanting to experience body positive, inclusive yoga. I was originally going to go with 'wholesome yoga' – but it sounded too much like a loaf of bread. I liked the word 'curvy' – but a quick Google search showed that all permutations of curvy were taken, or so I thought. Eventually, I decided to combine curve + some = Curvesomeyoga. It felt right and the rest, as they say, is history.

The goal of Curvesomeyoga has always been to ensure that the world of yoga is more inclusive and to encourage individuals who would not normally consider practising yoga to give it a try. I want everyone who walks into a Curvesomeyoga class to feel welcome regardless of his/her shape or size and be able to enjoy the transformational and healing benefits of yoga. Classes are in a judgement-free environment, where students have agency over their bodies and can work towards learning self-acceptance and self-love, inhabiting their bodies with more ease and comfort. They can choose to do as little or as much as they want – I always let students know that if they want to stay in Savasana (dead body pose) and breathe for the entire class that is fine. But most importantly, I want to allow them to feel part of a community that is welcoming – to enjoy a similar experience to mine. The philosophy is simple:

We are a body lovin' absolutely accepting space. All genders, shapes, sizes, ethnicities, age and levels are welcome. Wear what you like, be who you are; you are amazing just as you are right now and I want to help you feel comfy in your skin.

Practitioners initially come to yoga for a multitude of reasons, but they invariably gain so much more than they ever imagined. This really is the magic of yoga and I cannot say it enough: it really is for everybody!

Body positivity and diversity

Fast-forward to the present, and I've noticed the paradox that as yoga has grown in popularity, the less diverse it has become. My first yoga teacher was South Asian, my next was of mixed heritage, and I was able to attend a yoga studio owned by two Black yoga teachers. I took this for granted at the time and didn't realise how significant this was and that it would become an anomaly in the future – to be taught by and share this practice with teachers of colour. I could not have wished for a better start to my yoga journey.

During my life, it would appear that I had been blinkered, even though I experienced discrimination. As my journey has evolved, I see more and more areas where marginalised communities are not being invited to be at the proverbial table; many of us are now starting to create our own tables.

In 2019 I was invited to be a panellist at an event called 'Black Women in Fitness'; it was an amazing, but rare, experience to be in a room where people who looked like me were in the majority. Events like these are so few and far between that they always stand out for me. Being in a room full of Black women coming together to share their professional and personal experiences of being in wellbeing spaces was so enlightening. I came away with the realisation that there was a real need for safe, judgement-free spaces for the Black community.

This eventually led me to co-create NoireFitFest, to encourage more of the Black community to experience health and wellbeing while also showcasing the talents of the Black wellbeing and fitness professionals. I still can't believe that in 2020 it was the UK's first Black wellness and fitness festival. It was a success and demonstrated that events like these are much needed. The feedback was amazing – in 2020 it was Zoom-based because of the pandemic, but over 200 people attended online.

Yet again, this example demonstrates how yoga has allowed me to come home to myself. It has given me the strength to shift from merely assimilating to finding my voice so that I can become a good ancestor for future generations, just as the many good ancestors before me have allowed me to be Donna Noble (also known unapologetically as the Noble Yogi). Although the changes I would like to see may not all happen in my lifetime, I hope that I'm laying down foundations to ensure that future generations' wildest dreams become reality.

I am tired of waiting to be invited to sit at the proverbial table; instead I'm starting to build my own space and inviting allies to join me. We can't expect those with power to change. But we can start by being the change we wish to see in the world – by starting that tiny ripple we'll soon create the tsunami required for real change to happen. I'm not sure where this journey will end, but I will certainly try to enjoy the ride. I have some amazing allies who are helping me to do so, and I thank them.

A note on language

The language used within any environment is important, but even more so in a body positive class. I have chosen to use certain terms when referring to body types in order to create a safe environment where offence will not be caused:

- curvy
- abundant
- plus size
- bigger body.

I do not have the right to identify bodies based on my perception. I appreciate that some terms may be triggering or cause harm. As yoga teachers we need to be respectful and sensitive of the way individuals self-identify or self-describe.

The word 'ob*sity' is censored in recognition that some people may find it triggering.

2

What Is Body Positivity?

The history of the body positive movement

The body positive movement has become increasingly popular in recent times, but there is confusion over the meaning of the term. Very simply, body positivity means different things to different people, and the aims of the movement have evolved over time.

The oldest form of body positivity began with a campaign started primarily by a group of middle-class feminists between the 1850s and the 1890s. The Victorian dress reform movement, also known as the rational dress movement, set out to break the trend of women modifying their bodies. At this time, women were expected to wear extremely tight corsets to achieve the societal standard of a tiny-waisted, hourglass figure. This practice began during childhood and many Western women participated despite, unsurprisingly, finding it hugely uncomfortable. They also had to endure being criticised or mocked for achieving the abnormally tiny hourglass figures. Wearing tightly laced corsets also led to adverse health outcomes, as they caused women's ribs to become deformed and their spines to misalign.

The dress reform movement also argued for women to stop hiding their bodies underneath layers of fabric in the form of elaborate dresses and advocated for women's right to wear trousers. Although we might take the latter for granted nowadays, I remember having to campaign to wear trousers at secondary school during my time as school council representative. Maybe I was already a feminist and a little bit of a rebel even then.

We should also note that many middle-class women were beginning to go out to work at this time. It was also becoming fashionable for them to become healthier and more active, leading to the need for practical clothing, such as bloomers. In the late 1800s, a New England activist, Lilly Miller, designed trousers to be worn under short skirts, permitting greater movement and freedom. As time went on, other movements such as the flappers in the 1920s and land girls in the 1940s continued to push against gender norms and what was deemed by society to be an acceptable 'body image' for women. These women were strong advocates for the acceptance of women's bodies, whatever their shape or size. It's inspiring to look back and see examples of women who rebelled against the damaging fashion trends of the day.

The body positive movement re-emerged in the late 1960s, this time pioneered by Black and lesbian women whose focus was on ending the culture of fat-shaming and discrimination against people based on their size or body weight. The movement, and the activism which followed, was intended to inspire as well as to celebrate, validate and show acceptance of fat bodies, while broadening the cultural definition of what makes an acceptable body. It was a movement by and for marginalised people, and created a space for those being ignored by society because of their physical appearance. Its strong message of self-love provided a safe refuge away from oppressive mainstream beauty standards.

In the US, this resulted in the creation of the National Association to Advance Fat Acceptance (NAAFA), a non-profit civil rights organisation dedicated to promoting and protecting the rights of fat people. Body positivity was just one element of the NAAFA's ideology. Having a body that was widely reviled and discriminated against and to love it anyway, in the face of constant cultural messaging about your flaws, was (and still is) a radical act.

The term 'body positive' emerged once again in 1996, through Connie Sobczak, a psychotherapist who had been through treatment for an eating disorder in her teens and the death of her sister Stephanie. She founded The Body Positive (https://thebodypositive. org) in honour of her sister, who inspired her work to help people to appreciate and learn to love their bodies and in the hope that her daughter and others would grow up in a new world.

The current state of play

Fast-forward to present day and body positivity is everywhere. Its current form emerged in around 2012, and initially sought to challenge unrealistic beauty standards before shifting towards the message that 'all bodies are beautiful'. This can be seen at the forefront of fashion. Plus-size models and celebrities such as Lizzo, Candice Brathwaite and Ashley Graham are finally being represented on the catwalk, in mainstream media and on the covers of magazines. The body positive movement has also evolved and extended to include men, whose body-image issues are just as complex as women's. For instance, invisible constraints associated with being male include not being able to discuss self-image, and being seen as weak when being vulnerable or showing emotions. Men may also feel they have to conform to unrealistic societal expectations in terms of their bodies, as seen in the buff, six-pack bodies shown in movies and within the fitness world. Is this partly why mental health issues and suicides are increasing in young males?

I am so happy to see that some quarters of the mainstream are starting to be more diverse in terms of marketing. At the beginning of 2021, the UK edition of *Cosmopolitan* magazine published an issue where the cover shows a diverse range of bodies accompanied by the heading 'This is Healthy'. Unsurprisingly, there was a lot of backlash and debate around this, stating that two images in particular promoted ob*sity, demonstrating how health is (incorrectly) determined by looks. This equates to policing women's bodies and trying to stipulate which bodies are deemed to be healthy. We see a lot of bigoted and stereotypical language, where being fat is associated with being unhealthy and lazy. This is ridiculous; there are plenty of thin people who are unhealthy, and it's wrong to associate bad health with size.

We are also now seeing a growing recognition and acknowledgement that the LGBTQIA community face similar body positive challenges to other communities. Inspiring individuals like singer/songwriter Sam Smith are sharing their body positive stories on social media, which helps create safe, judgement-free spaces for discussion.

Everyone has the right to feel accepted, seen and acknowledged, and it is great to see that this is happening.

However, there is a major negative to this popularity – over-saturation has led to exclusion, where marginalised and plus-size bodies are no longer core to the conversation. We are seeing campaigns being launched that centre on embracing our bodies and finding self-love and empowerment, but these same campaigns continue to perpetuate the narrow framework of Western beauty standards.

It is also important to remember that body positivity is not about pressuring people to feel positive and love their bodies 24 hours a day, seven days a week. These pressures will be further marginalising, and it is okay not to feel this way. Another key point to consider is that not all of us need body positivity in the same way, because not all of us would become socially unacceptable without it. If you do a quick search of #bodypositive on Instagram, you will mostly see thin white women displaying their slightly curvy thighs – in other words, you will see people who have 'socially acceptable' bodies. I am not here to disparage anyone. Most people will experience their own insecurities and body hang-ups, but I have used this example to highlight the evolution of the movement.

We must take time to acknowledge the presence of Black women, femmes and plus-size folks who paved the way for white social media influencers. There is no body positivity if there is no social justice for marginalised groups that don't have a voice or a platform to share that voice. Not all bodies are subject to the daily harassment, stigma, discrimination and bias that stem from the fat phobia that permeates society. This is why the social justice element of the movement is required – there is no body positivity until everyone has equal rights in terms of education, employment, housing, and so on.

A body positive movement rooted in disrupting the status quo and smashing body ideals helps us all. The problem is that when we make body positivity centred on all bodies, the ones that are most marginalised continue to be so while the bodies that are already privileged continue to take centre stage. If we remove the roots of fat acceptance from the body positive movement, we have lost the true essence of the uncommercialised body positive movement and its original intention.

Body positivity is more than self-acceptance, and I am seeing that those who continue to embrace it are taking a stand against weight stigma and diet culture. By doing so, they are continuing the legacy of fighting against the oppression and injustice that people who inhabit a particular body are subjected to. Just to clarify, these bodies have evolved to include, but are not limited to, Black, queer, trans, disabled and neurodiverse bodies. If you are not doing something to support and advocate for people in these bodies, then you are exploiting the body positive movement. The core lesson from being part of the body positive movement is that all bodies should be equal.

Diet culture has no place in the body positive movement because it completely contradicts it in terms of philosophy and beliefs. Please note that there is a distinction between weight loss and diet culture.

YOGA AND DIETING/ANTI-DIETING

Diet culture is markedly different from weight loss. Weight loss is a personal endeavour and is undertaken for a myriad of reasons that may or may not have anything to do with the society we live in – however, I must state that weight loss and dieting is so normalised that most people would find it bizarre if you weren't on some form of 'diet'.

Diet culture on the other hand is viewing thinness as a moral imperative; Western culture is built upon and preoccupied with thinness or the Eurocentric beauty ideals.

From birth we are surrounded with overt and subliminal messaging that promotes being thin, from children's cartoon characters, to aeroplane seats being made for thin bodies and everything in between.

Diet culture is the unfortunate and harmful trope that you can be anything you want, just don't be fat – because then you'll be viewed as the worst kind of human.

> This has ramifications that are far wider and much more detrimental for all humans, but especially those who are fat. They are denied jobs and healthcare, and sadly treated as sub-human.
>
> *Aisha Nash, Anti-Diet Yoga teacher*

Some individuals are trying to reclaim body positivity, but fear that it will be an uphill battle as it has been so co-opted by the mainstream who believe, through no fault of their own, that the movement is solely about self-love. I see so many people stating that they are an authority but are in fact spreading misinformation and perpetuating inaccuracy. We need to acknowledge that self-love is not linear.

As for most historical movements, the roots of body positivity have somehow become distorted and changed to suit the current climate. My hope is that the body positive movement will evolve but retain its roots, and that the Black femmes who created it don't feel excluded, which is very much what is happening right now.

What does body positivity mean for yoga?

Body positivity is a game-changer for yoga. It can make a fundamental difference and dismantle some of the inherent stereotypes prevalent within Western yoga today. Most importantly, awareness around body positivity means that yoga is becoming more available to marginalised people who have, until now, been bystanders and felt unwelcome within the yoga space. It's also providing teachers with the tools to share their gift with anyone who wants to access yoga and try something that they've previously been excluded from. Through body positivity we can learn how yoga is a reflection of life and how it can help change the world, one yoga class at a time.

Learning about body positivity has changed the way I teach yoga and given me a better understanding of how to achieve my goal of making the practice more accessible and diverse; to appreciate that there's so much more to the practice than the asanas, and that the goal is not to get my leg behind my head, as in that image of Madonna that was instrumental in getting me started on my yoga journey. Body positivity has enabled me to take yoga off the mat and make it more accessible through social justice and creating equity.

We still have to ensure that body positive yoga is not entirely co-opted by the mainstream in the same way as other movements. Already we are beginning to see signs of this in the use of the body positive hashtag on social media. When you look this up, you'll see there's no evidence of true body positivity – it's fast becoming just another marketing gimmick to sell classes, clothes, and so on.

True body positivity is when everyone is welcome on the yoga mat. You can do this by creating a space where people feel empowered to let their practice accommodate their body and do yoga in a way that feels good for them, so they have agency over their body.

Body positivity means you and your body may be okay today and the following day, or perhaps not. Loving your body is far from easy, and it's a journey that may take time; accepting your body and all that it does for you as it is and not trying to change it is the core message. One of the things I try to get my students to do is to trust their body – because they do not even realise that they don't, having lost the connection.

I hope that those working towards reclaiming the body positive movement are successful, so that it continues to include and honour those who it was meant for, so that the fight for social justice can continue. My attempt with this book is to show that we can all be the change we want in the world, and for me, this starts with yoga.

3

The Roots of Body Positive Yoga

Body positivity throughout yoga's history

Yoga is a mind–body practice that is steeped in Indian philosophy. Its journey from its origins thousands of years ago to the current day has been a long one, and its many iterations have resulted in several different schools and styles of yoga. It appears that my journey has evolved just as yoga itself has!

Yoga has a diverse and rich history and there are many opinions on its evolution, especially regarding how it has been embraced by Western practitioners. Ironically, this practice, which was so diverse in its beginnings, has become less diverse as its popularity has increased. Yoga's rise within the mainstream means it's often compared to (and confused with) other forms of exercise and movement practices. The hope is that this evolution means that more individuals will begin to experience yoga in some form, that it will become available for the many and not the few. However, often only one element of yoga is seen – the asanas (postures) – and it can be accompanied by a competitive mindset, which many people find off-putting. Many feel that yoga currently perpetuates the view that certain body types are better than all others, but this was not always so.

Along the way yoga has become co-opted to the point where it's now unrecognisable to those who grew up with its teachings and has become inaccessible due to its commercialisation and appropriation. However, there is a movement that is working towards honouring the roots of yoga and making it accessible to all. This has social justice at its core. Like many, I believe that the practice should be rooted in philosophy, equity and unity. I am so pleased to see that yoga is being reclaimed, and its true essence is once again being shared so that the real benefits can be experienced. I wonder what the Brahmans and old masters would think of yoga's evolution. Would they be proud or disappointed?

The origins of yoga by the Noble Yogi (aka me)

My introduction to the history of yoga did not include many indigenous or traditional references and had a very Western perspective, although I was taught that yoga originated thousands of years ago in the Indus Valley. In my teacher training, one of my main reference points was the book *The Yoga Tradition* by Georg Feuerstein (1998), which formed part of the recommended reading list back in 2009 for my yoga teacher training.

The practice of yoga is thought to date back to pre-Vedic Indian traditions, possibly in the Indus Valley civilisation around 3000 BCE. The original yogic texts were written in Sanskrit, an ancient Indo-Aryan language that is the classical language of India and of Hinduism and considered to be one of the oldest languages on Earth. Sanskrit is also believed to have healing powers, which is unsurprising considering the healing and transformational benefits of yoga.

However, in 2012 I discovered a little-known fact – there is evidence that yoga has African influences, and there is a form called Kemetic yoga (also known as Egyptian yoga). Some people are now of the opinion that yoga started in Africa, a view that is beginning to get recognition within the mainstream yoga world (Ashby, 2006).

I didn't know about this form of yoga until I attended an audition where one of the other teachers demonstrated Kemetic yoga. The class really stood out for me as I'd never experienced it before. Although my curiosity was piqued back then, I didn't think about Kemetic yoga much until many years later, when I was asked about it during an interview on a local radio programme during Kwanzaa. (Kwanzaa is an annual celebration that was created in the aftermath of the Watts riots, to give African Americans an alternative to the religious and capitalist Christmas celebrations.) I'm afraid to admit that my knowledge was limited back then, and I couldn't talk with any real understanding of the subject. However, as my practice and teaching have grown, so has my knowledge, which I'll share with you now.

KEMETIC YOGA

Kemetic yoga is a yoga system based on the principles, philosophy and science of ancient Egypt, similar to what we commonly understand as yoga based in Indian traditions, but with a focus on geometry and the tongue connection. It involves a combination of physical movements, deep breathing techniques and meditations. It has a large emphasis on breathing patterns, the philosophies of self-development and self-discovery, and the healing of mind–body–spirit.

The physical postures are known as Thef Neter or Sema Paut, which represent the gods and goddesses (neter or neteru). Although these are important, the Kemetic practice emphasises activating the parasympathetic nervous system to create conditions whereby the body and mind can heal themselves. This is different to the goals of some forms of commercial yoga, where the main focus is the asana.

Kemetic yoga was known as Smai Twai, which means union of the two lands (i.e. upper and lower Egypt, relating to the physical land mass, or higher and lower self, relating to our spiritual being). Smai is also symbolic of the breath/union of the lungs, so we can see its relation to yoga, which derives from the root 'yuj' and is often translated to mean union or yoke. The word 'yoga' was not generally used in this way in Sanskrit.

Interview with Amani Eke, Egyptian yoga instructor

The people of ancient Kemet practised a unique style of yoga that some say predates and influenced the practice and philosophy of yoga in India. Images that date back some 10,000 years have been found on temple walls in Egypt, and these hieroglyphics and ancient Egyptian art portray people in poses that are typically seen in modern-day yoga classes. It would appear that there's been a rich dialogue between Africa and India for thousands of years! (Kemetic YogaSkills, n.d.)

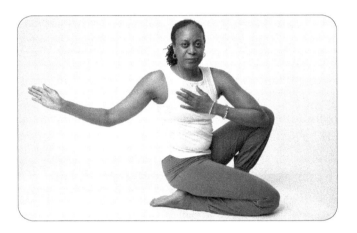

I don't profess to know exactly where yoga originated or whether the oldest form of yoga came from India or Africa – information is out there for those who wish to explore this further. There are arguments and debates about which came first, but I believe that we should appreciate this indigenous knowledge as a way of furthering the evolution of yoga. I believe that bringing attention to Kemetic yoga is good, and I would not have done this book justice if I hadn't taken this opportunity to highlight it. Bringing it into the mainstream offers an alternative perspective and a way to encourage more people to access a form of yoga that resonates with them.

My knowledge is based on the yoga training courses I've attended, but in recent years I've been enquiring into my learning as questions come up and trying to relearn in order to achieve a greater understanding of what yoga means. I realised I need to challenge what I took to be the truth after seeing how yoga has been commercialised in order to become palatable for a particular consumer. For example, I used to say that yoga is a 'lifestyle', but very recently I've realised that lifestyle is about privilege. I would even now start to say yoga and wellbeing is becoming a privilege for those who can afford it. The COVID-19 pandemic has emphasised the vast differences within society – not everyone has the luxury of choice; sometimes the fundamental thing is survival. This has made me even more determined to evolve and ensure that I try to offer a style of yoga suitable for everyone.

In this book I want to acknowledge that many cultures have potentially contributed to this great science/philosophy and that this diverse history should be embraced and celebrated. Isn't discovering Kemetic yoga another way of discovering the truth, just as yoga itself is about finding the truth of who you are so that you can be your authentic self? We can all find our own truth and practise in a way that resonates with our beliefs. This is a great opportunity to exhibit how one of yoga's main goals can be achieved, in the form of union.

Was yoga always inclusive?

I believe that we are all natural-born yogis. 'Happy baby' pose so eloquently proves this – have you seen a baby lying on their back with their big toe in their mouth? Bliss!

During my research, I discovered that yoga has always been inclusive in terms of accessibility and different body types, and there are numerous stories to substantiate this claim. For instance, yoga props are not a new phenomenon, and were originally used to make seated poses comfortable (Powell, 2018).

Although it would appear that yoga was initially primarily practised by men, the number of female yoga adepts (masters or experts who have attained a specific level of knowledge in doctrines) may have been considerably higher in India's past, when Tantra was more commonplace. Acclaimed yoga scholar Georg Feuerstein writes in his book *The Yoga Tradition*, 'Allama Praphudeva [a tantric yogi from the Natha tradition] was a contemporary of Basava (1120–1168 CE) and the head of an order that included three hundred realised practitioners, sixty of whom are said to have been women' (cited in Bell, 2018).

Another example is the story of how Astavakrasana (eight angle pose), which we might think of as an advanced yoga pose, was named after someone with physical disabilities who demonstrated that this did not prohibit him from benefiting from yoga – see the box below.

ASTAVAKRASANA (EIGHT ANGLE POSE)

Astavakrasana is an asana with an interesting history.

Once there was a great king called Janaka, who ruled the kingdom of Mithila and was the father of Sita, wife of Lord Rama. In Mithila there was a great sage called Uddalaka. He had many students learning under him, and one of the best was Kahoda. Uddalaka was so pleased with Kahoda that he gave him his daughter Sujata in marriage. Even after the wedding, the couple continued to reside in the Ashram of Uddalaka, where Kahoda assisted his father-in-law in teaching.

In time Sujata became pregnant. She would always sit near her father and husband while they were teaching. Her unborn child attained mastery over the Vedas by listening to his grandfather. One day Kahoda was teaching his students and his heavily pregnant wife was sitting close by. Kahoda was tired physically and mentally and made a number of mistakes while reciting the scriptures. Unable to bear these errors, the child started correcting them from his mother's womb!

Humiliated before his disciples, Kahoda cursed his son, saying, 'As you insulted your father, may you be born with eight bends in your body!' Accordingly, the child was born with his body crooked in eight places, and was named Astavakra (asta – eight, vakra – crooked). His father never loved him and never taught him anything. But Astavakra listened to everything his father and grandfather taught to their students and also learnt on his own.

One day a great scholar came to King Janaka's court and

challenged the scholars there to a debate. Kahoda went to the palace for the debate. When Astavakra realised that his father was not in the house he asked his mother where he'd gone and Sujata told him. Astavakra wanted to see the debate! He was very young (some texts say he was 12 years old, while others say 16 – I tend to think he was 16) and severely disabled.

By the time he reached the palace the debate had just finished, and his father had been badly beaten by the scholar. The arrogant scholar asked if anyone in the court could challenge him. Young Astavakra rose and told him that he would take the challenge. Everyone looked at him and started to laugh! Astavakra told the king, 'King, you are a great king! Please give me a chance. I can defeat him.' He gave his permission and Astavakra defeated the scholar easily.

Now Astavakra went closer to his father, knelt down and touched his feet in respect! Kahoda had watched his son during the debate with tears flooding from his eyes. He hugged his son and asked him for forgiveness while his tears washed over Astavakra, blessing him. Suddenly Astavakra's disabilities were gone.

Yoga teaches us that the body is the temple of the soul and we must take care of it. But if you become too concerned with the physical aspect you can cross that line and become obsessed with your own body and that of others. We should never judge the soul by what the body can do, or how it looks. Astavakra's story reminds us that yogis can come in all shapes and sizes and can be any age! Astavakra, even with his disabilities and without his father's love, became a great yogi.

In our journey to enlightenment, we will come across many obstacles, some of which can be very severe. Sometimes we must overcome our inner demons (like ego, attachments, ignorance), but a true yogi can overcome these obstacles with dedication, discipline and determination.

Mano Subramaniam, Yoga teacher

What does yoga look like today?

The true essence of yoga has been lost, leading to the exclusion of the majority of our society from being invited onto the yoga mat. We need to remember that yoga does not discriminate, not that you would think so by the way in which it's portrayed today.

As part of a quick experiment, I did an image search for 'yoga'. The result was pages and pages of pictures reflecting a stereotypical person who practises yoga: young, slim – often white – women in gymnastic or contorted poses. There was a distinct lack of diverse body types that were representative of our society in terms of shape, size, colour, ability and gender. It is shocking to see how white the Western yoga landscape has become considering its origins, as well as how few people recognise this. Is this because people don't get it or because they don't care?

Mainstream yoga has become a reflection of the fashion industry, where 'thin' is the ideal body type, and wearing on-trend clothes, having the latest brands and expensive equipment has become a prerequisite for practice. I saw this for myself when I first started Curvesomeyoga and exhibited at the Om Yoga show back in 2015. I was shocked to find out that I was the only exhibitor – out of hundreds – who was catering for anyone over a UK size 14.

For many, how yoga looks has become more important than how it makes you feel and its transformational benefits. When I started practising yoga back in the late 1990s, I was wearing a mismatch of workout/gym clothes – and these were sufficient. No one cared or even noticed what I wearing and I was accepted just as I was. It was only when I was preparing to attend my teacher training in Los Angeles that I became aware of 'yoga fashion', and was often being told that I needed the right yoga clothes. Not wanting to be the odd one out – I obliged. Nowadays I'm still confident in wearing what makes me happy. I appreciate that being a yoga teacher does unfortunately mean that I get judged on my appearance, but I am no longer defined by that.

All of this immediately presents a barrier to certain sections of society getting on the mat. Although things are starting to change, there's still a long way to go. Why would you consider engaging in an activity if you perceive that it's restricted to a certain group of people? Representation and imagery are important, and these examples highlight the role they can play in making yoga appealing to those who need it the most – often the marginalised and invisible members of our society. Progress towards diversity is further hindered by the front-of-house staff at yoga studios or gyms often conforming to a particular stereotype. Then there is a continued lack of diversity in the changing room itself, where students often feel daunted. There are so many minefields to navigate before even getting on the mat. Then, when students who are brave and resilient enough finally get there, they don't feel welcome in the room or feel safe. Accessing yoga should not be a constant battle.

'You can't be what you don't see' is a phrase that I have started to use often, simply because it's so true. Representation matters. If the imagery we see doesn't reflect our society, why would someone even entertain the idea that yoga is for them if they cannot see anyone who looks like them? It all makes perfect sense and is something that can be easily rectified. An example of this comes from my own experience. I was at the Om Yoga show in London and had a conversation with a woman – I'd assumed she was a little curious about yoga as she was at the show, but she was adamant that yoga wasn't for her. By showing her a picture of Jessamyn Stanley (who looks similar to this woman), I could convince her that she too could do yoga.

How often do you see a picture of a yogi of colour or with a curvy body doing yoga? It's so rare in the vast majority of mainstream media that it often appears to be an anomaly and sometimes brings about negative reactions. For example, when *Cosmopolitan* UK had Jessamyn Stanley on their front cover they received an alarming amount of negative coverage about her health. These assumptions were based purely on looks, with no medical information whatsoever to back them up. Thankfully, we have inspirational yogis like Dianne Bondy, Jessamyn Stanley, Anna Guest Jelly and Dana Falsetti who have shared their practice online, showing that yoga can be accessible for all. It is so wonderful to see practitioners of different shapes, sizes, genders, ages and ethnicities showing the world that they, too, have a yoga body.

Instagram and social media

I have a love–hate relationship with Instagram and social media. Like many things, social media can empower and educate in a positive way, or create comparison in terms of the information and the images that are shared. It was an essential part of allowing me to challenge the status quo and it allowed me to follow amazing accounts and create a community. As with anything, we need to filter what we absorb. I try to ensure that I am not triggered by any information being shared; if I am, then I simply unfollow. Your social media is a reflection of you and your values. It is also a platform where you can share your values.

Although it perpetuates the kind of mainstream yoga imagery described above, Instagram's visual nature also means that it has empowered so many individuals to share their practice and can be a tool to effect change. It's so exciting to see so many yogis sharing their practice online so that they can record their yoga journey. This in turn inspires their community, who see the transformational benefits of yoga and are encouraged to challenge the stereotypes of who can practise it. This creates the much-needed diversity that is currently missing from the yoga world, although the abundance of what are described as 'yogi Barbie' images still means such diversity is overshadowed.

Unfortunately, it's not always possible to show the many facets of yoga in a single post – so what you usually see is an asana (posture), which invariably is a pose that looks unachievable for most people, like an arm balance or a complicated inversion. Why not Tadasana (mountain pose) or Savasana or seated postures? Why do we think that difficult poses will encourage individuals to want to practise yoga? This non-inclusivity and overt exclusivity shows that the individuals unable to achieve the tricky asanas are not welcome within a yoga space. As yoga teachers we are in many ways the 'face of yoga' and should share content responsibly. Next time you post something to your account, why not try to be creative and show more accessible aspects of the practice, like meditations or breathing exercises? I recently shared a picture of myself in Balasana (child's pose) draped over a bolster and I received the comment 'I felt a jolt of co-regulation just by seeing the picture'. This goes to show that simple postures can be more effective in welcoming practitioners to yoga – so we are able to invite and include the many and not the few.

Allyship

Greater representation of different groups practising yoga in the mainstream is really refreshing. Although awareness is growing across the board, this seems to be short-lived. One example is #BlackoutTuesday on Instagram during June 2020 (shortly after the death of George Floyd) where brands and influencers posted a black square with a promise not to post anything else during the course of the day. The intent was for those taking part to show allyship and diversify their content, while reminding non-Black people to reflect on how they may benefit from racism. Those black squares disappeared very quickly. It was trendy for a day or two to pledge support but it soon went back to business as usual.

Time has passed and there have been some changes but it's not enough. The wellbeing industry needs to be held more accountable for its lack of diversity in a sustained way. I appreciate all the individuals who amplified and shared my voice on their platforms so that I was able to share my lived experience with their communities. However, at the same time a lot of lip service was displayed with little or no long-term action. The overall landscape doesn't look very different – I have certainly been on the receiving end of performative allyship, where individuals or organisations claim to advocate for a marginalised group but don't back this up with actions; however, instead of accepting this when it occurs I 'call it out' – not always publicly. I do this so that others will not have to endure a similar experience and so that brands are not able to plead ignorance.

A similar trend happens during Pride Month in the form of 'rainbow-washing' – the act of using or adding rainbow colours and/or imagery to advertising, apparel, accessories, landmarks, and so on, in order to indicate progressive support for LGBTQIA equality (and earn consumer credibility) – but with minimal effort or pragmatic result. (This is akin to 'green-washing' with environmental issues and

'pink-washing' with breast cancer – see www.urbandictionary.com.)
We're seeing more and more rainbow flags during this period, but
where is that support and visibility during the remaining 11 months
of the year?

Allyship is a continuous process and it is not always easy or quick
(and is certainly not a sprint). Ask yourself, 'How am I supporting
communities that do not have a voice?' The question I ask is where
is everyone who posted the black squares and what have they done
to continue to support the Black community? My hope is that it does
not end up the same way as the #metoo campaign, which received a
lot of coverage but was very soon forgotten. The same mistakes can
be seen within the yoga community where there are already signs of
tumbleweed and things have gone back to business as usual. We are
still seeing discrimination of people in the form of ageism, sizeism,
colourism and sexism.

Are your actions of inclusivity performative allyship?

As the Black Lives Matter movement surged into global consciousness in 2020, a large percentage of diversity has been performative,
resulting in tokenism. Take, for example, the black squares people
posted on Instagram. The message behind this became diluted and
got somewhat lost. At that time, my inbox was full of brands who
were eager to work with me, giving the (false) impression that they
were allies; however, their only purpose seemed to be to want to
avoid being called out and to steer clear of the issue so that they
wouldn't be held accountable.

Performative allyship is where someone in a privileged position
vocalises their solidarity with a cause. This allegiance is then used to
distance themselves from scrutiny. This is a trend that is continually
being reported on and I should not be surprised by this, but I will
continue to call it out.

I do have a positive personal example of allyship. A yoga friend
was asked to write for a well-known yoga publication. She was
asked to contribute an article, but what she did instead was to
recommend yogis of colour, including me, providing us with an

opportunity to amplify our voices. Being an ally does not mean that you have to march in the streets, but it does mean you can consider using any privilege that you may have to support the communities that need it.

I was so touched and grateful for this gesture. In light of everything that took place in relation to Black Lives Matter in 2020, she went on a personal journey of discovery and learnt more about what she could do to use her privilege to help others. She took the time to read the book *Me and White Supremacy* by Layla F. Saad (2020) and completed the exercises so that she could discover and dig deeper into her privilege. She also read other recommended books and did the exercises, even though sharing her experiences and talking about diversity lost her followers on Instagram as this wasn't something she normally shared with them. That did not deter her, and did not matter to her as much as being a true ally. I wish that there were more people out there like her. I urge you to be one of them.

Inclusivity is at the heart of yoga

People come to yoga for many reasons: it is trendy, friends are talking about it, it has been recommended by medical practitioners, or just plain curiosity. They might even have certain goals in mind, possibly to become more flexible, regain their health or be less stressed. This will be achievable, but people are often amazed when they are able to gain so much more. That's the beauty of yoga – you expect so little but it can in fact be life-changing. I am an example of this. Saying that yoga is a journey may sound very clichéd, but it really is. It's the journey from our outer into our inner world, where we really start to connect with the essence of who we are, which sometimes gets buried beneath social expectations and the conditioning of our formative years.

The purpose of yoga is essentially to have your own individual experience. We can all be doing the same poses, but each person will experience them in their own way. The asanas may even look different, as they will reflect our own unique bodies and interpretations of what we're doing.

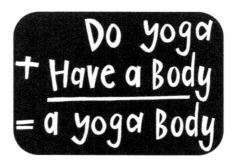

I really believe this to be true, and have been proven right time and time again. The classes I teach can vary: sometimes students will be diverse in terms of different shapes, sizes, ethnicities, abilities and ages, while at other times they reflect the Google search result and lack diversity. Even in my own class I can still be the only person of colour. I'm okay with this, as I understand that there is still a long way to go in terms of creating greater diversity in the yoga room. I like to teach to the bodies that are in front of me and ensure that the students allow the pose to fit their body and not for their bodies to fit the pose.

Often students' ability is judged by the size of their body. I have experienced this, when it's been assumed that certain yoga poses would be easy for me to achieve but this hasn't been the case. Conversely, I've taught students who don't realise what their bodies can achieve. I always say that you should never judge anyone by their shape or appearance, as this can be very deceptive and lead to inaccurate conclusions and judgements. As individuals, we should appreciate the body for all the amazing things it does rather than focusing on what it cannot do.

Community is the aspect of yoga that resonates with me the most. The reason for this is that I've always wanted to ensure that *everyone* has access to yoga, and this has resulted in me creating communities that may not always be reflected in mainstream yoga studios. I firmly believe that yoga is only an advanced practice if there is a space available for everybody on the mat.

When we come together, we are able to enjoy the transformational benefits of yoga. Community is union in action, as we are all able to collectively experience yoga by sharing our diverse cultures. In turn, we can then gain a better understanding of how we should come together so as to make this world a better place, eliminating divisions. Through being on the yoga mat, we have an opportunity to learn first-hand about each other so that we can bring this knowledge into our everyday lives. By developing a more informed insight to diversity we can embrace differences.

The true essence of yoga encompasses so much more than just the physical element of the practice. Allowing the ancient teachings to be core to our practice means there is hope of spreading more love, compassion and awareness to ourselves and others. Let's allow our practice to be the basis for all that is good and be compassionate.

When the true meaning of yoga is understood it can bring about connection and social justice, as witnessed within the eight limbs of yoga (see Chapter 11). Yoga is the gift that keeps on giving.

.

Part 2

CREATING INCLUSIVE CLASSES

4

What Is a Body Positive Yoga Class?

A body positive yoga class is where yoga is taught in an inclusive and accessible way for every body regardless of shape, size, ethnicity, gender or dis(ability) within a safe, judgement-free environment.

When body positivity and yoga blend it results in inclusive spaces that allow students to feel empowered and where we as teachers challenge the way in which society views and uses the physical body. The normalisation of all body types within the yoga space helps students to find freedom within their body and their practice. The main goal is to create an affirming environment that allows students to have agency and the ability to advocate for their own individual needs. Essentially it is about body sovereignty, where students are able to feel safe within their body.

The student is always in charge of their body and experience. It should never be about the teacher. The students know their body best – in fact they are the experts, their own gurus. They know how the posture feels in terms of good and bad sensations so can avoid harming themselves. Sometimes they may require a little encouragement, as they may not be aware of their body's full potential – something I've experienced myself on numerous occasions. All bodies are unique and should be treated that way.

There is a positive focus on abilities, not disabilities. In life it is easy to focus on the negatives rather than the positives, and this can be felt both on and off the mat. Focusing on disabilities can create a barrier between student and teacher and can result in the student deciding to stop practising.

A body positive class is the complete opposite of the image of yoga currently portrayed within the mainstream. Students will be accepted just as they are and it will be acknowledged that everyone's yoga may look different. The focus is less about achieving perfect alignment and working towards 'beautiful' postures and more about what's happening internally. It's about feeling the postures from the inside out so that a mind–body connection is created. At its core, the message is one of self-acceptance and a belief in oneself.

The pace of the class is slow, to accommodate everyone's needs. This gives each student sufficient time to find a variation that's suitable for their body, including the use of props. It also provides them with the time to observe and feel the pose and experience its benefits. This means that students are unlikely to injure themselves, and can connect with the breath and slow down the movement and their thinking so that they can be more mindful (so that they do not feel lost or confused). There are so many health and mental benefits. I love to witness students starting to trust their body, to discover their body's true potential and as a result realise that they are so much more than how their body looks, becoming empowered in all aspects of their lives so that they are able to navigate this world in a happier and healthier way.

Classes should be fun and without expectations – falling out of postures should be normalised and students should be encouraged to take a pause or reset whenever they want to. Give them assurances that there's no need to try and be perfect. It's about yoga practice and not yoga perfect. Every time they get on the mat, it will be a different experience. Sometimes my own practice may be strong and focused; other days it's shaky and distracted.

Attending a body positive class should not be about the students trying to strike a pose like me or mirror the teacher's body in terms of achieving each pose. It should be about accommodating their body in a way that allows the pose to be executed in a way that resonates and feels good for them. Variations are offered to cater for the different bodies and abilities, and props are an essential part of class as they enable accessibility (see Chapter 8). These are not to make the postures more challenging, but to offer a different way of doing the pose.

Teach poses in stages. Actually *teach*. Don't just *show* what the pose could look like; break it down. What's stage one? Stage two? Stage three? Work these out for yourself. If a student can't do stage one, find something that they are able do that will help them to get going. The aim could simply be to allow the students to feel comfortable within a variation of the yoga pose that suits them. As well as having an awareness of the various body types of the people who come to my classes, it's also important to eliminate the hierarchy of postures that are primarily taught in traditional yoga classes, where we are taught that the pose will eventually lead to what some call the 'full expression of the pose'. I like to think of my yoga mat as a yoga lab – which gives me the opportunity to be creative and really dissect the poses so that I am able to make them accessible. I try, where possible, to teach all poses, even those that may be considered challenging, as there is invariably a way to make them accessible. It should also not be assumed that a body positive yoga class is a beginner's class, as it will evolve with time. It is a class that will have students at different stages of their yoga journey.

THE BUS STOP METHOD

One way to bring different options for poses is the bus stop method, which was introduced to me on my training with Dianne Bondy and Amber Karnes. Different options are offered, and the students are able to get off the proverbial bus at a stop that is appropriate for them. For example, in Vrksasana (tree pose):

Bus stop 1
Balancing on one leg, placing the toes of the other foot on the floor or on a block.

Bus stop 2
Placing the foot on the standing leg, below the knee.

Bus stop 3
Placing the foot on the standing leg, above the knee.

We'll talk more about appropriate language in Chapter 6, but be aware that absolutely no diet talk should take place in a body positive class. As well as being triggering, it's an inappropriate subject to bring up, as I'm not a qualified nutritionist. There should also be no talk about achieving the infamous 'bikini body' or fitting into a 'little black dress'. All bodies are celebrated and accepted.

Creating a body positive yoga class

There are a number of steps you can take to create body positive classes.

- Ensure that you recognise and work to remove unconscious bias.
- Educate yourself on accessibility by attending trainings.
- Continually assess your classes to make sure they are inclusive.
- When advertising your classes, be sure to clearly articulate what you are offering so that people's expectations are met. Is your beginner's class really for beginners?
- Take steps to create a safe space for all.

Recognising unconscious biases

Unconscious biases are social stereotypes about certain groups of people that individuals form outside their own conscious awareness. Everyone holds unconscious beliefs about various social and identity groups, and these biases stem from one's tendency to organise social worlds by categorising. It is important to note that biases, conscious or unconscious, are not limited to ethnicity and racialised identity. One's age, gender, gender identity, physical abilities, religion, sexual orientation, weight, and many other characteristics are subject to bias.

It should be known that we all have unconscious biases or blind spots. Biases can be so ingrained that people aren't even aware of them. They're a cause for concern, but the real issue is when people are in denial about them. As teachers we need to do the work of self-study so we can uncover any of our own potential biases and where possible challenge our assumptions (see Office of Diversity and Outreach, n.d. for more information on unconscious bias).

UNCONSCIOUS BIAS

Affy Uffort told me of her experience of unconscious bias:

'I had a photoshoot with a lovely photographer and the pictures were so amazing. I was absolutely proud of myself. However, another yoga practitioner/teacher made a comment insinuating that I was overeating because my body was not typical of what yoga was about. In her words, "Yoga is not overeating or being overweight. I really like this way of encouraging people to practise, but this is not what yoga is."

'She didn't stop there when challenged by others. She added that my picture instead would inspire those who are overweight, which is something good, but that if I was really practising it would be impossible for me to stay as overweight as I am, as yoga requires one to gain control over all your addictions, including eating habits. So literally without knowing me she had come to the conclusion that I was overweight, I had an addiction, and I wasn't practising yoga because I wasn't as skinny as she was. It was a bit disappointing to witness such unintelligent thoughts and words. People's mindsets need to change, and they need to support each other from a place of love and elevation.'

This is a perfect example of unconscious bias and how it can create harm. The other teacher made a judgement about Affy's health status based how she looks and nothing else. This is wrong on so many levels. As teachers, we need to ensure that we don't unintentionally cause students to feel unwelcome or triggered when they walk into the yoga room.

Training

Accessibility should be a core principle of yoga, but unfortunately it's not covered during most 200-hour teacher training courses. This means that most new teachers have little or no experience of teaching diverse bodies or communities. That is certainly my personal experience too. I would advise seeking training, which is what I did when I started to think about offering body positive yoga classes, as I didn't feel I had the relevant experience. I had no hesitation booking onto Dianne Bondy and Amber Karnes's Yoga for All online training course in 2015. It gave me the confidence to ensure that my classes were accessible.

In addition, I completed the Accessible Yoga training with Jivana Heyman and subsequently assisted on the next training in London. I also attended workshops with Jessamyn Stanley and Dana Falsetti, among others. These trainings inspired me to be creative in my teaching and showed me how to share yoga with those who are missing from the yoga space. I'm not an expert on all of these topics, but investing in training has made me unapologetically unafraid to pioneer change within the wellbeing world. A highlight was when Jessamyn generously donated her time in hosting a Q & A session I organised about body positive yoga back in 2015. The feedback from all the attendees was amazing. Here's a link to the session: https://youtu.be/BilmdlmrTTA.

It is great to see so many teachers becoming part of the movement to change this narrative, and long may it continue. However, on these trainings there was a lack of diversity in terms of age, size, ethnicity and gender. I was often the only person of colour, and at this time the ideal of the 'yoga body' was already starting to be cultivated.

As yoga became more Westernised, we began to see the idea of the yoga body, and social media added impetus to this. To evolve, we need to continue our learning and education. I recently realised that the training I unconsciously make reference to most and that had the greatest impact on me is my hot yoga training; I'm not sure why, but it had a profound effect on my journey. Maybe this is partly due to its diversity. There were trainees from approximately 28 countries, and I was able to interact with teachers from different walks of life who wanted to share the transformational benefits yoga had for them. Practising with and learning from teachers from around the world, which would not have been possible previously, was a privilege and one of my best experiences.

Having access to more online training courses means that there is now greater opportunity for trainings that are diverse in terms of teachings and participants. It is good to see that an increasing number of mainstream teacher training courses are introducing diversity and inclusion modules within their training.

Evaluating the accessibility of your classes

The COVID-19 pandemic has meant that there are more yoga offerings online, but we need to remember that this doesn't automatically equate to greater access. Some people may not have access to a computer or Wi-Fi, and not everyone finds working with technology easy. It's good to see that there are accessible and inclusive classes that have been created to ensure that all communities are catered for; for example, yoga classes where sign language is available for those who have impaired hearing.

What steps are you taking to ensure that no one is being left behind? When we communicate online, are we taking into consideration that English may be some students' second language? What other factors could you consider to make your classes as accessible as possible?

Later in this chapter, we'll cover some of the other barriers to people accessing yoga classes and some ways to help overcome them.

Describing your classes clearly

Ask yourself, 'Is my class description clear?' For example, so many students sign up for beginner's yoga, but find when they attend the class that it's for students who already have a yoga practice, resulting in them not returning or being completely put off from returning to yoga. Always put yourself in students' shoes, or try to remember your first ever yoga class and how you felt. I appreciate that attending a yoga class can be one of the most daunting things ever. I've had students sign up and pay for a class but then feel so much anxiety about what to expect that they don't show up. Sometimes this is because of all the misperceptions about yoga and the way it's portrayed.

Students need to feel that attending a yoga class will be one of the best decisions they will make, and should have no regrets. I often say to people that if they have any fears or anxiety about attending a class they can talk to me beforehand, or even attend and observe it with no obligation.

My first experience of yoga was when I was at university; I joined the campus gym and gave a few different classes a go. I liked the essence of it, but I always wanted to try yoga as I'd seen so many people talk about how much they loved it. It wasn't until a few years later that I went to a yoga class, but I walked out really disappointed that it hadn't lived up to expectations. The class was far too quick, despite being billed a beginner's class, and I didn't feel any benefits whatsoever. It didn't put me off trying yoga again but it definitely could have.

Tara Tomes, PR expert and entrepreneur

Creating a safe space

Students are making themselves vulnerable to teachers when they come to classes, and they need to be treated with the respect and love that they deserve. We don't know a student's path to yoga or how much effort it has taken them to do something that others may take for granted.

I've personally found imagery to be an excellent way to provide potential students with a sense of what attending my class will be like. How can we expect someone to attend a yoga class if they are not convinced that they belong in the first place? This is especially important for students who may be excluded or feel excluded from the mainstream (e.g. those who don't have the mythical 'yoga body'). As discussed in Chapter 7, more diverse yogis are using social media to share their practice, meaning that body positive yoga practices are being shared more than ever before. This is really good to see. You can also use these channels to make your students feel welcome in your class before they even step onto the mat (see Chapter 6). Another option is to offer newcomers a free taster class so that they can experience your energy and see the type of community you've created. Signing up for a 4–6-week course may seem like a daunting commitment, so a taster is a great way to demonstrate that your class could be beneficial to them.

Challenges of teaching body positive classes

Creating an inclusive class does not come without certain challenges, and I will address some of the ones that I've encountered along the way.

If I had waited or not had the encouragement to start creating inclusive classes I doubt that I would have created Curvesomeyoga. I almost talked myself out of it on so many occasions. I was also still the proverbial 'new girl' in the yoga world, so who was I to think about offering something different? Well, I'm pleased to say that my imposter syndrome was eventually silenced and here I am now, writing a book about body positive yoga. I would have laughed if this had been suggested back in 2015!

One of the first challenges I encountered when starting my body positive journey was the pushback I received from friends who could not believe that I had created Curvesomeyoga and said that I couldn't teach curvy bodies, because I was not curvy. I was stunned by that reaction, and initially thought they were right. However, I soon had the determination and courage to continue after speaking to another friend, who noted that you don't have to be gay to advocate gay rights, so why not teach yoga to people with curvy bodies? As a Black woman, am I limited to only teaching yoga to people that look like me? My thinking at the time was that it's better to have someone offering these classes, no matter what they look like – and no one else appeared to be doing so.

There were also times when I first started teaching when I would be challenged by the various body types of the people who came to my classes. It was a steep learning curve, but what I learnt was not to be discouraged by a body that was different from those I had exposure to during my first trainings, and work with the body and the pose instinctively, ascertaining what the pose was trying to achieve rather than focusing on how it looked. It was during this time that I learnt about being creative, and if necessary being open with the students and letting them know that I didn't always have the answer. They would often understand – I believe it showed them that I was human and not perfect. However, I ensured that I would go away and research and come back with an option for next time. As mentioned previously, it was the various trainings that provided me with the confidence and skills to be able to grow as a teacher. This is one of the reasons that I try to keep my classes small and treat them like a workshop so that I am able to help and serve as many students in the best way possible.

Students will have their own criteria for selecting yoga teachers, and I certainly know that my looks and size will prevent me from appealing to some. For example, if they have a choice of two teachers, some students are going to select the one that looks like them, and this is understandable. I know and appreciate that such choices are made because it's assumed or felt that the teacher will understand or encounter some of the lived experiences of the student. However, I'm pleased to say that the vast majority will not make this their primary consideration.

When looking for a teacher, I would actually look for someone who looks like me; a bigger girl, full of confidence, loving yoga and moving her body in an unapologetic way. I think it's so helpful to have a more diverse selection of teachers out there; someone who 'gets' it and also brings together a similar group of people. Especially in the early stages, if you're still building your confidence, I think being surrounded by people who have a similar level of ability and, likewise, similar challenges is really crucial to help you keep going. This means that the teacher can better serve you all, but it's also great when you see someone relatively similar to you pushing themselves and achieving great things.

Tara Tomes, PR expert and entrepreneur

Another argument I heard against introducing body positive classes within the London yoga community was that creating specific classes would cause division – yoga is all about union. This even went as far as questioning whether there was even a need for body positive/ inclusive classes, because the general classes were already inclusive and welcoming to everyone. There are pregnancy and women-only classes, so what is wrong with having classes that help ensure every-body has access to yoga? By seeing me overcome these objections, those very individuals have changed their minds and seen the value in creating these environments. In an ideal world, there would not be a need for such spaces, but that moment has not arrived (yet!). I am pleased to say that I'm no longer challenged in this way.

Teaching mixed levels/abilities

As yoga continues to evolve, we will hopefully see more mixed-level/ability classes where everyone feels empowered to make yoga their own and practise their own version of it in a single class, using a chair, mat or (as I call it) Paul the wall. I have been fortunate to have the opportunity to teach mixed-level classes at my local community centres and at workshops. However, it should be noted that teaching in this way is not always embraced in mainstream studios by all students (see the section 'Debunking myths about props' in Chapter 8), and this environment may be off-putting for people with diverse bodies.

Teaching mixed-level classes does have challenges, but with practice it becomes easier and provides us as teachers with the opportunity to create classes that are accessible to a wide variety of yogis and for growth. I discovered the art of teaching mixed-level classes during my Accessible Yoga training. Before this, I wasn't aware that it was possible to teach classes in this way, but I quickly realised that this is how I wanted my classes to be: where nobody is left behind, and where an option is available for everyone. I came away from the training with such enthusiasm and hope for being able to create these classes and spaces.

Some teachers do not believe that it's possible to teach different bodies and abilities in one class. I understand that some yoga schools don't acknowledge the use of props, and there are teachers who adhere to this mindset rigidly. But with a growth mindset, lots of practice and the proper knowledge, it is indeed possible to create these classes. I'm hearing from more and more colleagues who have been able to achieve this.

Remember – yoga is always evolving. The image of yoga that I saw during my teaching did not include curvy bodies, people of colour, mature bodies or bodies of different abilities. So why would I or anyone else believe that this could be challenged? The same can be said for mixed-level classes. With access to information and training and the move to make yoga more accessible, more teachers are starting to feel better equipped to teach students of all body types who might enter the room.

Here are some tips for teaching mixed-level classes:

- If it's an established class, teach to the majority of students in the form of cueing, but demonstrate for those who wish to do variations that they feel are suited to them. For instance,

I start the class using the chair, so the students can choose whether to use a chair or not.

- Always adjust the way that you teach to suit the majority – so if your room is 80 per cent beginners, teach to them and offer options for the rest of the class. I usually provide three variations of each pose and then say it's 'yogis' choice' as to which option is practised.
- Be approachable. This will allow students to feel able to ask questions and also avoid students being reluctant to do the poses or feeling left behind, confused or frustrated.
- Talking to your students before class is the best way to determine the combination of levels you'll have in your class, especially if it's open to all levels. Alternatively, you could use regular students to help welcome new students so they do not find the class too daunting.
- When teaching an inclusive class you must try not to lose the engagement of the whole class for just one or a small number of students. One great way to do this is to introduce 'yoga playtime'. This is a time (for which I normally allocate between two to five minutes) where students can become playful and practise any poses they are working on. So you can have a room where some students are in Balasana, and some in Bakasana (crow pose); it's their choice. This is an excellent way to accommodate all levels of students in an inclusive way.

Barriers to accessing yoga

Sadly, there is an endless list of barriers that prevent people from accessing the transformational benefits of yoga. In order to understand why some people feel that yoga is not for them, we first need to understand the barriers they face. By understanding the challenges that face our students we can help to create truly inclusive classes. Some of the challenges I have seen are:

- The need to make space for the body – some body parts (e.g. the stomach, breasts, etc.) can obstruct the body from being comfortable in a certain position; for example, breasts getting in the way when doing Salamba Sarvangasana (shoulder stand).

- Feeling their bodies do not look like the others in the yoga space. I recall a student saying that they always occupied the same spot in the room because they were conscious of the size of their butt and didn't want to have someone standing behind them. We should therefore not always make judgements about attachment to a place in the room as this can be deeply rooted. The teacher should allow the student to practise where they feel comfortable, but may wish to investigate why there is an attachment after the class.
- Being body shamed. This is something that I did not expect to experience, but I did – all because the mobility and flexibility of my body did not meet the teachers' expectations.
- Even in a body positive class, someone may be concerned that they may be the largest person in the room.

'I don't have a yoga body'

The image of yoga conveys that it is only practised by people who are tall, slim and white, flexible and female, with the 'ideal yoga body' and able to do advanced postures. As discussed elsewhere in the book, there's a distinct lack of diversity within the wellness space and the yoga industry. How can you expect someone to be what they don't see? Those from marginalised groups will often feel uncomfortable in yoga spaces because they feel invisible. Have you considered how we as teachers may inadvertently be contributing to this barrier? Take a moment to imagine what a mainstream yoga studio looks like and visualise what sort of marketing is used to advertise classes. Are these images really designed to appeal to everyone? Make sure to be aware of issues surrounding diversity and actively work towards welcoming diverse bodies to your classes.

I went to a yoga class today and at the end the instructor asked me why I want to be a yoga teacher. I said that I find that there are not a lot of yoga teachers in the area who look like me [gestures around belly]. The instructor grabbed her belly and said, 'We are out here.' This lady must have been maybe a US size 12 [UK size 14] at the most. I just kind of smiled and nodded uncomfortably but couldn't bring myself to really say anything else. I just need to say that it is so frustrating for someone who is barely plus size to equate their struggles to the struggles of people of much larger size. Representation matters, and this woman just did not get it.

Anonymous

'I'm not fit enough'

Although many forms of movement work from the outside, where the main focus is on aesthetics, yoga connects to the body from the inside out. I often say that yoga is essentially 'a work in and not a workout'. It is so much more than the physical postures. Some people are under the illusion that they must have a certain fitness level before even venturing onto the mat. It can therefore be really nice to offer relaxing and restorative yoga classes!

'I'm not flexible'

Flexibility is not a prerequisite for starting a yoga practice, but this does not stop it from being an excuse not to start practising. Increased flexibility can be a natural by-product of yoga – you will gain flexibility in both the mind and the body – however, beginners are not always aware of this. This misconception is caused by the image of yoga – seeing someone in a pretzel-like pose on social media and advertisements for yoga classes will make potential students believe that they need to be flexible in order to be a yogi. Instead of inspiring students to step onto the yoga mat, such images are having the opposite effect.

The original (or as I like to refer to it, 'old school') yoga mainly focused on sitting for long hours rather than contorting the body into a sequence of asanas. The aim was (and is) a focus on the breath and learning how to breathe, but this is often not communicated to prospective yoga students. Somehow the asanas have instead become the desired outcome of yoga for many. It's our job as teachers to remind students that flexibility in asanas is not what yoga is all about; understanding the principles of breathing and how other aspects of yoga can be taken into everyday life is where real yoga can begin.

Yoga class locations

Where are your classes? Are they located in the areas of the population that you wish to serve? We've seen that mainstream yoga studios are often in affluent areas, primarily where there is a demographic that will be able to afford to attend yoga classes. I've seen this as areas have become gentrified, which inevitably results in the arrival of yoga studios. Seek out new possibilities for reaching different, less affluent communities in order to make classes more accessible. However, when students find classes that provide them with the ability to relax and find enjoyment, distance is not always a barrier. If you create a safe, judgement-free environment, you may find that your students will travel to experience it.

During the COVID-19 pandemic, teachers and studios have had to dramatically adapt to teach online. I believe this has resulted in the empowerment and financial independence of some teachers, who could fit teaching around their other commitments and become more connected to an international community of teachers and trainings. In some instances, teaching your own classes online rather than in a studio means you can teach in a way that resonates with and is authentic to you, so it's something to consider when making your classes available to different sections of the community (for more discussion about the benefits of teaching online, see Chapter 12).

What times are your classes?

There seems to be a trend for free yoga and beginner's yoga classes to be scheduled at off-peak times, when the studios are least busy.

As businesses, studios will schedule the most popular classes at peak times, but these may not be suitable for beginners. We need to remember that some yogis interested in accessible classes might be working or have childcare constraints. The yoga landscape and people's habits have changed as we emerge into the 'new normal', so now might be a good time to gauge interest – especially with the hybrid model of in-person and online classes.

'I don't have time to practise yoga'

Another objection I've heard is that yoga takes time and people don't feel they have sufficient time to practise. However, the opposite is true: yoga creates time. Let's look at this in a little more depth – time does need to be allocated for yoga practice, but one of the benefits is that you become more focused and efficient, so the end result is that you gain more time. I personally find that it takes me longer to leave the house without practising yoga because I spend time searching for mislaid items (keys, mobile phone, etc.) due to my lack of focus. My practice allows me to be more prepared and able to remember where these things are, thus I save time because of the investment I made in my practice. It provides the mental clarity to organise life more efficiently, which results in becoming more productive and reducing activities that hold you back.

A yoga practice can be a little as ten minutes a day. As I always say, 'some yoga is better than no yoga'. The feeling you experience once you have finished your practice is so worthwhile. Before you know it, by the end of the week, you've completed 70 minutes of yoga. Once this becomes a habit, I've found it will invariably become longer, and once you start to see the rewards and benefits in your everyday life you can't stop.

Religious connotations

Another common objection I hear is that 'yoga is religious', but yoga can be whatever you want it to be. We can worship whomever or whatever we want and can also decide to dedicate our practice if we wish, to whatever or whomever resonates with us; this could be the universe, ourselves or someone/something we care about, or God. I always give my students the choice to do this. The beauty of yoga is that it's a very individual and personal practice.

It should be caveated that there are some yoga schools that are devotional, for instance Bhakti yoga, which uses the method of attaining God through love, achieved through chanting the names of various gods. The goal is oneness with the Divine. It should be remembered that a body positive yoga class does not adhere to a particular style or school of yoga, so although the practices taught in a class will have the teachings, influences and beliefs of the teacher, students should have the autonomy to dedicate the practice to whomever or whatever they want or not at all.

I have first-hand experiences of misconceptions around yoga and religion. One example is when I attempted to hire church halls: in some cases my request was refused, and other times I've been asked to promise not to recruit the parishioners to yoga in the belief that I would convert them.

'The language is too complicated'

Some students think that yoga has its own language (and we're not even talking about Sanskrit). Students hear us say things like 'breathe into your back body' or 'lengthen your tail bone' and feel confused. When you first heard something similar at the start of your journey, did you understand it? Think about how you can use language to ensure that students can understand your instructions and intentions.

The combination of lack of knowledge of yoga poses and Sanskrit can overwhelm students. I know it's all part of the yoga journey, but I can understand this issue. To make things a little easier, using the English equivalent will make the practice more accessible. Personally, I use both the English and Sanskrit names when teaching body positive classes.

'I don't have the right clothes'

Is there a requirement for specific clothes in order to practise yoga? As I have said so many times before, the answer is an unequivocal NO! As long as students are comfortable in their choice of clothing, that's all that matters. They can wear whatever they want and so can we, as teachers.

'It's too expensive'

Yoga is everyone's birthright, but the cost of attending classes can be prohibitive. The price of a drop-in class in London can be in the region of £20 and over. Three classes a week comes to an eye-watering £240 per month. Even with a discount for multiple classes, that's inaccessible to the average person.

I believe that doing yoga is an investment in one's health. It's certainly helped me to heal mentally and physically. Making this investment in yoga has helped my health and saved money on the treatments (physiotherapy, etc.) that I no longer need. As we know, yoga is not a panacea, but it is often referred to as 'preventative medicine' as it can help us avoid potential future health problems; it's increasingly being recommended as a health self-management tool by some medical professionals, and a number have adopted social prescribing to prescribe yoga and other activities with health benefits.

WHAT IS SOCIAL PRESCRIBING?

In recent years there has been an increase in the number of doctors offering 'social prescriptions' instead of traditional medicine in order to help relieve the pressure on the already strained health services. Doctors are recognising that health is determined by a complex range of social, economic and environmental factors. Social prescribing has afforded the medical profession the option of referring people for a range of activities, such as yoga, gardening and other sports.

The aim of social prescribing is to empower people to have more control over their health, while also cultivating community to achieve a healthier and happier life. It addresses people's needs in a holistic way.

Yoga can and should be affordable and accessible. A potential way to make yoga accessible is by posting some free online classes on YouTube or another platform. Offering free content can be controversial, as it can impact teachers' salaries, but it's an excellent way to entice people onto the yoga mat.

I'm wondering if there's a compromise that will satisfy both sides of this ongoing argument. There are so many ways in which we can make yoga affordable and accessible to all.

- There are schemes and funding available that allow teachers to offer yoga and other activities for free to the local community. I successfully received funding from Sportivate and other organisations when I started offering body positive yoga classes.
- Karma classes are another option. These are usually offered on a donation basis and students are encouraged to donate what they can, knowing that 100 per cent of the proceeds of the class will go to a charity.
- Some students help out on reception or clean around studios in exchange for free classes. This is known as being a Helping Hand.
- Donation-based classes are another option, where students can pay what they can afford to attend. Yoga is seen as a gift and an education in some cultures, where teachers from these communities allow students to pay as little as £2.00 per class. Yoga is not seen as something that should be profited from.
- A pay-it-forward model is where a member of the community can purchase a class, workshop, and so on, and it is then offered to someone who would like to take the class but may not be able to afford it.

Accessibility issues

When I went to Berlin to attend the Accessible Yoga conference, I stayed in a hotel that was 100 per cent accessible. I remember Jivana Heyman asking why we don't have more accessible venues. As an ageing population, the majority of us will, at some stage, potentially have access issues or experience disability.

We need all venues and studios to have wheelchair access. Having ramps and lifts is the first step to making buildings accessible. I do understand that there are limitations in some cases due to size and building restrictions, but this should not be a reason for change not to happen or for efforts not to be made. There are only a handful of mainstream yoga studios that can welcome wheelchair users; I am lucky enough to be able to hire venues that allow me to cater for ALL students so that I can offer genuinely accessible classes.

Disability

Shortly after my training, I attended the Accessible Yoga conference, where Matthew Sanford gave a keynote speech via video link. He recounted a time when he was teaching a student who was paralysed, and their connection was so deep that it went beyond the physical; it was as though they touched each other's hearts. It was incredible, and this, in turn, touched me so much and reminded me why I teach yoga; it really is about the feeling and not about achieving a particular posture. The ability to communicate without words – to see beneath the skin we inhabit to connect to a person's soul – is a skill we need to lean into and develop as yoga teachers. When we withdraw from all the external distractions (the superficial) and make a connection in a profound way, this is where we see that we are truly all one. Is this when we achieve Samadhi (enlightenment)?

Yoga can be experienced by anyone, in any body, but many people will feel that having a physical disability may exclude them from practising. Bed yoga is one option to ensure that nobody is left behind and all bodies practising yoga are normalised. We're going to see classes like this more and more as a greater number of teachers make their yoga practice accessible.

We also have to remember that not all disabilities are visible, which is why we need to teach from a place of compassion or love – not forcing our expectations on our students. It will not always be apparent why the student is reluctant to complete a request. For instance, if a student decides not to remove their socks, accept this rather than allowing a battle of wills to ensue, as I have witnessed in class before. I remember a few days after becoming a certified hot yoga teacher, I was teaching a class in New York. I asked a student to release his index and middle finger in Kali mudra, which is part of the hot yoga series. At the time I thought he was ignoring my request so I repeated it – it was not until he showed me it was impossible that I realised my mistake. To say I was embarrassed was an under-statement – but a valuable lesson was learnt. If something similar occurs during one of your classes, you need to take time afterwards to investigate why this happened, so that you can appreciate the student's predicament and avoid repeating the situation.

Yoga as a 'lifestyle' can be off-putting

The popularity of yoga has now seen an increase in it being marketed as a lifestyle, but this can have negative connotations as it can be associated with luxury and wealth. I'd never considered this until another teacher I met during a training course outlined how lifestyle can be seen as a privilege that is taken for granted by many of us, and this exclusivity goes against the idea of creating union. This was a lightbulb moment for me, as I realised that this was yet another barrier that prevents students from starting their yoga journey.

The word 'lifestyle' is subjective in terms of how you incorporate the yogic teachings into your life. To stop idealising the yoga lifestyle we need to show the health benefits of yoga, ensure that affordability is not an issue and promote the fact that cultivating a practice is for everyone. Although mainstream imagery may make it look like you need expensive equipment (mats, clothes, etc.), we don't *need* all these things to start a yoga practice. Being vegan or vegetarian is also often associated with a yogic lifestyle, but these are just individual choices. Is yoga solely an exercise that involves you going to class every day because the practice makes you feel good, or just to hang out with your friends and be part of a community? Or does it go much deeper, when you start to incorporate the yogic principles of the Niyamas and Yamas and social justice into your life?

I have found that the more you incorporate yoga within your life, the more conscious and aware you become of how you treat your body. We have the opportunity to remind students how to take the teachings into their everyday life (either by challenging some long-held views or incorporating self-care, for example). A yogic lifestyle may creep up on you, starting first with a daily practice, then eventually consciously shaping your attitudes, your general way of life and your habits to be congruent with the principles, philosophies and ethics of yoga, to the point where you embrace the eight limbs of yoga. I prefer to refer to yoga as a journey that will allow you to discover who you are, because it is an individual experience, and your yoga is created experientially.

Why is it important to overcome these barriers?

I know that I keep saying that yoga is a gift, but it truly is a valuable tool that can help make this world a better place. When students come to us they are sometimes at their most vulnerable and want to start healing. Sometimes they don't even know what they want!

But whatever the case, we need to be able to create safe spaces and environments that help them to grow and heal and find their own path.

We can all argue and express our opinions about how yoga should be available. There will always be pros and cons; however, it's not always about us but about the students that we serve, and we must endeavour to give them what they want so that they can access health and wellbeing.

Our students are not our clients they are our students.

Dirish Shaktidas, yoga teacher

I love this quote for reminding me that we can adapt the yoga for our students too much, and thus lose the essence of the teachings.

Although some teachers naturally teach in a way that is body positive, it should be noted that solely calling a class body positive or accessible does not necessarily make it so. Preparation and training are required, and creativity helps.

5

Diversity and Body Positivity

Every body is a yoga body

When we say, 'every body is a yoga body' in the context of a body positive yoga class, we go beyond the definition portrayed by the mainstream yoga industry. The term 'yoga body' can sometimes imply that there is only one right way to look and feel if you practise yoga. Just like race is a made-up construct, perhaps we need to think the same about the concept of a yoga body. The term is considered by many to be a myth that limits the reach of yoga, and this is reflected in the lack of diversity within yoga spaces. In reality, however, there is no such thing as one perfect yoga body. *Every* body is a yoga body.

This is an image I commissioned back in 2015 when I first started my body positive journey. Upon reflection I can see that it could do with being updated as there are some bodies missing.

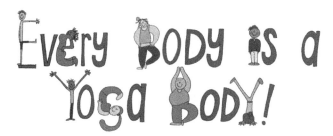

The phrase 'Every body is a yoga body' is now so ubiquitous it seems to be one of the most popular hashtags used by the yoga community to market classes. However, ironically, not *every body* is shown when you peruse the social media feeds; it's just a marketing gimmick.

All of this has led to the creation and maintenance of a hierarchy of bodies within yoga, with young, lean, flexible and able bodies, and proximity to whiteness (the list goes on) seen as more desirable and valuable, more in alignment with a yoga lifestyle or practice. The assumption here is that certain bodies are 'better', 'healthier' or more able to do 'advanced' yoga. The positioning of these bodies as aspirational is wrong on so many levels. Yoga itself is not the problem. The real issue is exclusion through biases, discrimination and lack of representation. It is the false notion of what a yoga body is, especially in terms of what we're now seeing in the association between yoga and fitness.

No one has the right to decide what a 'yoga body' is or define how it should look, especially if this definition is not inclusive. In its simplest form – if you have a body and are doing yoga, this equals a yoga body.

WHAT IS HEALTHISM?

The term 'healthism' was first coined by Robert Crawford in a paper for the *International Journal of Health Services* in 1980. It is now seeing a resurgence in the wellness and holistic health spaces. He defined healthism as 'the preoccupation with personal health as a primary...focus for the definition and achievement of well-being; a goal which is to be attained primarily through the modification of lifestyle' (Crawford, 1980, p.368). The system then defines health in terms of a person looking a certain way, and it also classifies behaviours and habits, bodies and foods as either 'good' or 'bad' based on whether they are perceived as being healthy. This is seen all the time within the fitness world, where fitness professionals (fit pros) determine someone's health based solely on looks.

The evolution of a yogi

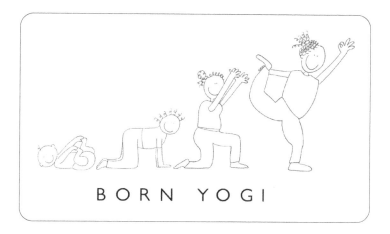

BORN YOGI

As I stated earlier, we are all born yogis – so by default I believe that we all have a yoga body. Before we know it, we are doing yoga; yoga is in everything. I would go as far as to say that yoga is everything: living, connection, finding balance, coming home to yourself, losing balance – we are yoga in action. At birth one of the first things babies do is take their first breath – this by its very nature is yoga. Have you noticed how naturally flexible children are? Often, they're doing poses like Vajrasana (fixed firm pose) while simply watching the TV. They don't care how the posture looks; they're only concerned with the way it makes them feel, they're so in tune with their bodies. If children continue to do yoga, they'll naturally be yogis, which will help them navigate this world and appreciate how amazing their body is. They already have self-acceptance of their bodies. If we lose our innate yoga practice (our natural abilities), we can regain some of the abilities we had as children if we start practising in later life. We can also lose our yoga when we start to adhere to societal expectations in terms of flexibility of the mind.

Yoga is a very personal practice; it's created through experience. This is at the very heart of body positive yoga. It doesn't matter how our bodies look when we do yoga; the most crucial thing should be how we feel. That's where we get to the depth of what yoga is. By saying that everyone has a yoga body and meaning it, we move away from the unhelpful definitions found in the mainstream media. The phrase 'yoga body' should represent all body types, all of which should be normalised, rather than the very narrow image we see at present. People of every shape, every colour, every gender, every ability, people in chairs, people in beds – they are all doing yoga in ways that accommodates their body.

Some teachers may feel insecure because they don't represent the mainstream image of how they believe a yoga teacher should look. When teaching body positive and diversity and inclusion workshops I am encountering more teachers who are questioning whether they should be yoga teachers because they don't feel they conform to the image of what a yoga teacher should look like. This is very concerning, because being a yoga teacher should not be contingent on how someone looks. This so sad to witness, and I try my best to be a reassuring voice so that they see that they have made the right decision and are good enough. Their worth is not based on their appearance. Remember, students will be attracted to your energy and will come to your class regardless of how you look. You cannot appeal to everyone, but being authentic will help you overcome your insecurities. It may not be easy, and may take time, but your confidence will grow as you begin to believe that you too are worthy and provide a representation of our diverse society. This certainly was my experience.

Representation matters, and is so important in all aspects of life, not just yoga; how can students be what they can't see? If by being visible you can encourage even just one person to try yoga, that is a great achievement – that is what I would tell myself in the beginning of my yoga teaching journey. The mainstream PR machine for yoga has done an excellent job of making yoga seem inaccessible and non-inclusive, and it is our job to undo this both for our students and for our community of yoga teachers.

One online campaign that I love is the Yoga and Body Image Coalition's 'This Is What a Yogi Looks Like' (#whatayogilookslike) (see Yoga and Body Image Coalition, 2014), as they do an excellent job of challenging stereotypes within the yoga community. This campaign is an effort to stand up to mainstream representations of who practises yoga, who should practise yoga, and what a 'yoga body' looks like. Yoga is more than a fitness trend. Yoga is a multi-faceted practice available to all.

Body image and yoga

We come in so many wonderful shapes and sizes, and this should be applauded – we are all unique. We are born into our bodies and take them for granted, not realising all the amazing things they do for us. Yoga presents us with a wonderful way to grow into and start to appreciate our bodies, and sometimes we only see them fully for the first time when we start a yoga practice. Yoga can be seen as a way for us to cultivate self-acceptance and self-love for our body. Again, this is a key component of body positive yoga.

However, this isn't always easy. Many people struggle with their own perception of their body, and their reasons for this can be diverse and complicated.

It is so important to remember that when you suggest that somebody should perceive themself and their body differently, those people with the most entrenched beliefs will be more resistant. So, asking them to change how they see themselves may more deeply inculcate the opposite view. Allowing yoga to organically give rise to change may in some cases be a more helpful strategy.

I know this, for on my own healing journey, even though body issues weren't my main problem, every time I was asked to create positive thoughts and aspirations, all it would do was make me think the opposite. When they would say, 'I love myself', all that I would hear is, 'that's not true, Heather. I hate myself.' It was much more about being with whatever was naturally arising, while doing the practice, that led to enduring changes for me.

Heather Mason, The Minded Institute

Participating in yoga can have a positive impact on body image because it:

- increases feelings of gratitude for our bodies
- improves self-confidence
- allows us to feel a sense of accomplishment
- can lead to positive physical changes in our bodies
- allows various body types to practise yoga together, thus normalising all bodies, rather than just a few.

The yoga mat is where you can find unconditional acceptance and self-love, one of the aims of body positive yoga. It's where the connection with our innate wisdom starts, showing that our worth is not defined solely by how we look. Discovering what is important allows us to let go of the things that are not serving us well (people, jobs, thoughts or possessions), leading to a happier and healthier lifestyle, while also relieving stress, anxiety and mental health issues. Yoga has been identified as one of the best ways to bring the work of body acceptance from the mind and integrate it into the body, an important part of the process. It can very literally bring you home to yourself, so that the body's true potential can be achieved.

I like to consider yoga's value in improving body awareness from a neurological perspective. We could talk about teaching people to love their bodies, question their thoughts and become more comfortable in their bodies, but I think that we can have very enduring negative self-talk, and I am not sure a yoga class is going to alter that; this is the work of deep therapy. If we look at Streeter *et al.* (2012), we get a picture of how yoga alters body perception through practice that leads to neuroplastic change. The researchers suggest that the practice of yoga increases GABA, the main inhibitory neurotransmitter in the brain, and that over time this leads to shifts in brain structures associated with perception of body state, such as the insula. GABA, via increased vagal input to the brain, is being released at high levels, rewiring the insula in conjunction with the prefrontal cortex; this then leads to an organic shift in perception.

I believe that with this shift in perception, where there is more congruence between one's perception of the body and objective reality, one may divest beliefs about the body that cause suffering and develop a greater sense of esteem for the body. I'm not saying this definitely happens, but I think this physiological mechanism may explain some of what many report occurs through their practice. Notably, at the same time you're releasing all these other neurochemicals that are improving your mood, and so when you put these all together, I think that you are becoming more accepting of who and what you are.

Heather Mason, The Minded Institute

Body shaming can take many forms. It occurs when someone makes derogatory comments about or criticises someone else based on their body shape or size, either to their face or without their knowledge. It also happens if you criticise your own appearance through comparison with someone else. Regardless of how body shaming arises, it often leads to lack of compassion and negative feelings towards one's own body. It has no place in the yoga space, but unfortunately I have experienced this first-hand on a number of occasions. I recall being body shamed while in a hot yoga class. We were about to go into Prasarita Padottanasana (wide-legged forward fold), but as a result of having tight hips, I could not separate my legs as widely as the teacher wanted or maybe expected me to. He stopped teaching the class and said, 'We won't move on until Donna opens her legs wider', which was virtually impossible given my body's limitation. On another occasion, where I was part of a class that was being photographed for a local studio, I recall the teacher looking at me in Baddha Konasana (cobbler's pose) and saying in front of the entire class, 'Your hips are bad and they are worse than mine' (she certainly laboured the point). I felt very self-conscious as I became the focus of the entire class, and remember being made to feel embarrassed about my body… It ruined the rest of the class for me. I'm sure the teacher did not realise what she was doing, and I don't think that she realised that she was body shaming me. But this is a perfect example of body shaming and how NOT to teach yoga.

Mental health

Mental health, defined by the World Health Organization, is 'a state of well-being in which the individual realises his or her own abilities, can cope with the normal stresses of life, can work productively and fruitfully, and is able to make a contribution to his or her community' (World Health Organization, 2018). Negative body image is now being associated with increased risk of some mental health issues, which include eating disorders and depression.

Using yoga to help with healing and mental health issues

Mental and physical health are very closely allied, but also essentially equivalent – there really is no health without mental health. Yoga is becoming an appealing way to deal with stress and to better manage numerous symptoms and conditions. There is increasing scientific evidence (NCCIH, 2021) that yoga is a great approach for overall health, and it is now being viewed by health professionals as a potentially helpful approach in a patient's recovery for various mental health issues. Some other issues relevant to body image and mental health include:

- long-term health conditions
- cultural differences around body ideals
- gender and sexuality.

Yoga is bio-psycho-social and we know that the approaches that work with the biology, the psychology of a person and their social interactions are quite potent. The eight limbs of yoga also match really nicely with the bio-psycho-social paradigm as they focus on self-reflection and behaviour, breath, movement, mental development and connection.

I think that yoga is such a potent strategy because you're working with the physiology at the same time as practitioners are cultivating self-awareness. The philosophical teachings of yoga are also supportive. You are teaching people that they're not innately unwell, that there is an inherent part within them that is always mentally healthy, but that certain faculties of mind have been cultivated at the expense of others. Beneath all of this is an enduring luminous self that is always accessible (albeit with effort) and never tainted by the ebbs and flows of the mind or life. When you help embed this belief while there is also juxtaposed a changing physiological landscape, I think you have the scope for profound transformation.

There was a time when we thought that yoga would be beneficial primarily for depression and anxiety, and not for more acute conditions like eating disorders, psychosis, schizophrenia and other conditions where psychosis is a major feature, borderline personality disorder, substance abuse disorders and post-traumatic stress disorder (PTSD). However, as more research is conducted, we are finding that yoga practice is beneficial for almost every mental health condition that we look at. It should be noted that not all of the research is robust, and so we cannot take each finding as a stamp of success. The best evidence for yoga's efficacy is for depression.

Heather Mason, The Minded Institute

The benefits of yoga are plentiful and numerous, and so we are now starting to see it being prescribed by some of the medical profession. Therefore, the chances of you teaching a student who has come to class in search of healing is higher than ever before. You may not, however, always know what issues a student is experiencing as they may not be immediately obvious, or the student may not tell you. Yoga teachers therefore need to be equipped with the tools to deal with students who are turning to yoga as a way to heal and find help.

Yoga is considered one of many types of complementary and integrative medicine approaches. As it brings together physical and mental disciplines that may help people achieve peacefulness of body and mind, it can help them to relax and manage stress and anxiety.

Mental health and eating disorders

An eating disorder is a form of mental illness characterised by an unhealthy relationship with food. This may be in the form of eating too much or too little food, and becoming obsessed with your eating patterns. One study found that even brief exposure to media messages portraying an 'ideal body' was linked to increased body-image concerns and increased disordered eating symptoms (Loeber *et al.*, 2016).

I recommend that all yoga teachers take an eating disorder course. It is a really valuable thing to do. Courses on yoga for eating disorders are available through Eat Breathe Thrive (www.eatbreathethrive.org/yoga-and-eating-disorders-free-short-course) and The Minded Institute (https://themindedinstitute.com/yoga-for-eating-disorders).

We need to note that anyone can develop an eating disorder, regardless of age, gender, size or ethnicity. Just like yoga, eating orders do not discriminate.

Body shape and yoga

For me, all bodies should be normalised, and I don't hold one particular body type in higher regard than another. When I teach yoga, I meet the students where they are, because I have invested in training with teachers that allow me to teach diversely, acknowledge my students as individuals and provide them with a yoga practice that works for their bodies. I would like to say that I do not see size.

However, this statement could easily be misconstrued, in the same way that some people say, 'I don't see colour.' When I hear people say this, it makes me think that they don't see me or don't want to understand my lived experiences. The fact is that I am treated differently because of the colour of my skin, just as many people are treated differently because of the size or shape of their body. If you don't see colour, then how can you see and acknowledge me and all that I stand for? By claiming not to see size, am I failing to acknowledge the lived experience of someone in a larger body who feels that they have not been able to take up as much space as they wish, both on and off the mat? I understand and appreciate from my own ordeals that all experiences matter. I love this journey, as it challenges our thinking and ensures that we adapt.

The world appears to be designed to accommodate a small percentage of the population, rather than the majority. For example, many clothing stores only stock certain sizes, and aeroplane seats are not designed for people above a prescribed body size. In yoga terms, many classes are not taught in a way that accommodates different body shapes, leading to those with curvy bodies not feeling welcome. If you reside in a curvy body, then you are penalised. The price paid for this unfairness can be high in emotional terms. Although I hadn't always realised or acknowledged this because it didn't often impact on me, an awareness of it has always been there, despite being buried away.

The characteristics of our bodies can contribute to our behaviour. I've heard reports of curvy individuals being asked to move to the back of the room in yoga classes, and fellow students moving their mats away from them. Students in curvy bodies often try to make themselves smaller so as not to attract any unwanted attention, because of the types of reaction they endure due to their size or appearance. This is why one of the first things I do in class during Savasana is to invite students to take up as much space as they like – so that they can let go and release any tension or stress that they are unconsciously holding in the body.

Many aspects of body shape vary with gender; the female body shape, especially, has a complicated cultural history and is based on societal standards that are subjective and vary between cultures.

Throughout the research for this book, I saw that a particular body type is being promoted (in the yoga sphere and in society in general), which adheres to societal norms. But recently we have seen the evolution and expansion of the number of terms and categories by which people may be identified.

Different identity characteristics

As body positive yoga teachers, we need to appreciate all forms of diversity. We have numerous identities that define who we are and which need to be acknowledged and understood. Our identities have a profound role in our lives – for instance, they can preserve tradition and provide connection with our ancestry. There's so much information to unpack around the role that social identities play in our lives in terms of how we show up in the world or are seen through different lenses. We are all truly unique and I genuinely believe that differences should be celebrated and embraced, as they contribute to making the world a better place. The world would be a boring place if we were all the same.

Two flowers next to each other never compare themselves, yet they are able to bloom – this way of thinking needs to be brought into the yoga space. In a body positive class, all students of all backgrounds are welcome, but as we have seen elsewhere in the book, not everyone will feel that they belong in the yoga space, because of the limited ways that yoga is represented. They may feel that they don't have the right body shape, or that only people of a particular race or culture practise yoga. It is our job as teachers to be aware of our students' feelings about this and do what we can to reassure them that the yoga space is for all. Below, I outline some of the different identity characteristics that may affect how your students experience the world.

Gender

The term 'gender' refers to the characteristics pertaining to (and differences between) women and men in terms of masculinity and femininity that are socially constructed – cultural differences rather than biological ones. Recently the term is used more and more to denote a range of identities that do not necessarily relate to the established ideas of male and female. These characteristics may include biological sex or gender identity.

In the last 12 months, I have noticed that general awareness surrounding gender diversity has increased. For example, chosen gender pronouns (e.g. her/she/he/him/they/them) are often included in people's bios on various platforms like Instagram and LinkedIn, and on Zoom. The thinking behind this is to allow people to express their gender identity if they wish to, but also to normalise this expression – if cisgender people show their pronouns on their profile, the hope is that it will make all groups feel safer to do so. In some instances, this information is being requested as a default on trauma-informed yoga courses. However, we need to be careful to ensure that individuals are aware that revealing their pronoun is not mandatory – it's a choice. There may be a number of reasons why someone does not wish to identify with a pronoun or disclose it, or is unsure how they wish to identify. I've witnessed first-hand that some people don't feel comfortable revealing their pronoun. When students sign up for my class they complete a health questionnaire, where they are able to add their pronoun (if they so wish). Likewise, individuals should have the right to decide their own gender identity and not have to conform to a rigid and outdated belief system. More information can be found at MyPronouns.org, Gender Construction Kit (genderkit.org.uk) and Gendered Intelligence (https://gendered intelligence.co.uk).

GENDER FLUIDITY

Although the concept and experience of a third gender is only recently coming into the Western mainstream consciousness, in many different cultures and spiritual traditions around the world there has always been an acceptance, understanding and even reverence for people who do not simply identify as being men or women.

In her book *The Spirit of Intimacy: Ancient Teachings in the Ways of Relationships*, respected healer, teacher and elder Sobonfu Somé shares wisdom about the Gatekeepers among her community: the Dagara people of Burkina Faso. She states that 'Gatekeepers are people who live a life at the edge between two worlds – the world of the village and the world of spirit...':

> The Gatekeepers stand on the threshold of the gender line. They are mediators between the two genders. They make sure that there is peace and balance between women and men. If the two genders are in conflict and the whole village is caught in it, the Gatekeepers are the ones who bring peace. Gatekeepers do not take sides. They simply play the role of the sword of truth and integrity. (Somé, 2000, p.132)

This reverence from the community and need for insight from the life experience of people that celebrate both genders within themselves can also be seen in other parts of our world. Among the following cultures, third-gendered people are also called upon for their connection to Spirit in some way:

- In Hawaii, Māhū people (who can be male or female at birth) are understood as third-gendered people. They hold traditional, spiritual roles, educating their society about ancient sacred traditions and rituals.
- Among First Nations people of North America there is a Two-spirit Zuni tradition. Two-spirit people live as embodiments of masculinity and femininity and are often looked up to as mediators, priests and artists.
- The Incas of South America would pray to Chuqui Chinchay, an androgynous, dual-gendered god. The Incas also respected their third-gendered people as shamans and healers.

Similarly, the role of non-binary people is seen among Samoans, who respect the Fa'afafine of their community, and the nomadic Chukchi people of Siberia, who also recognise a third gender. In these cultures in particular, third-gendered people play a big part in the family unit, often responsible for raising children, as well as hunting for their families.

Bringing it back to yoga and Indian spirituality, there is a deity worshipped within the spiritual tradition of Shaiva Tantra called Ardhanareeshwara. Ardhanareeshwara is depicted as half Shiva (the divine masculine Lord of Awareness) and half Parvati or Shakti (the divine feminine Goddess of Energy and Power). As a queer person who loosely (but lovingly) holds the identity of being a woman, it has brought me great comfort to see both Shakti and Shiva within myself. I love to embody both masculinity and femininity in the way I dress, move my body and relate with others. For me, being open to both within myself makes my experience of life richer and keeps me in a state of curiosity about what I do not yet understand about being a man and also about being a woman. Non-dual Shaiva Tantra has helped me to understand life as a constant flow between divine masculine and divine feminine energies. Both are needed within all beings in order to create insight, harmony and balance in our universe. To over-emphasise or reject one is to create toxicity and not honour these two distinct creative forces which made us.

Ava Riby-Williams, community facilitator and yoga teacher

Sexual orientation

Sexual orientation is a person's sexual, romantic and/or affectional attractions, to persons of the opposite sex or gender, the same sex or gender, or to both sexes or more than one gender. Examples of identities include heterosexual, gay, lesbian, bisexual and asexual.

It was a few years into teaching yoga before I felt comfortable to come out at my yoga studios. It wasn't that anyone was openly homophobic or biphobic, but I didn't see any allyship so I didn't know what the reaction would be or if it would be safe to come out. As a bisexual woman, it was easier to let people assume I was straight. It's only been in the last couple of years, in which I have created specifically LGBTQIA yoga classes, that I have felt able to bring my full self into my teaching and the communal aspects of a yoga practice. It's been life-changing.

My clients have also told me how much of a difference they've found being in a space where they know that all of their intersecting identities are not only tolerated but celebrated. This is particularly true in classes like pregnancy or postnatal yoga, which are so often full of assumptions and gender stereotypes: even the huge assumption when stepping into that space that you're a woman, you're married to man, and he is the father of your child. It's still common in so many pre/postnatal yoga classes.

Gabi Parkham, yoga teacher and
LGBTQIA equity educator and consultant

Ethnicity

An ethnic group is a group of individuals who share traditions, language, cultural heritage, nationality and ancestry. It goes beyond physical characteristics to traits that you share with the culture around you. For instance, some of my shared cultural characteristics are language, practices and beliefs.

Culture

Culture encompasses the behaviours or beliefs, practices and characteristics shared by a group of people. I demonstrate my Jamaican culture by wearing my hair in styles like braids or locs (a style where hair is sectioned into small segments and twisted, then left to grow), or through my love of Reggae music. Acknowledging this identity is important to me as it enables me to identify with my ancestral heritage.

Racial identity

Race is an invented, fictional form of identity; a social construct that has nothing to do with biology. It was created by European colonisers to legitimise domination and inequality and protect advantage. The concept of race still shapes our experiences, and our outward appearance is used to read us as a particular race. The physical features a group of individuals may have in common include, among others:

- hair colour
- eye colour
- facial structure
- body structure
- skin colour.

Many people will experience discrimination or face stereotypes due to their racialised identity, which can be extremely emotionally damaging. This has resulted in me having to be aware of how I behave when teaching, for fear of being accused of being 'the angry Black woman' when all I am being is assertive.

Intersecting identities

All the above help us to identify who we are, or are not, as the case may be. I am aware that there are many intersections of identity, and these can determine how our life is experienced. Let me use myself as an example: I am a Black woman and I am discriminated against based on the colour of my skin *and* my gender. My body's ability – whether I am considered healthy and able to do certain things – is judged purely in term of how it looks. I will experience the world around me differently to a Black man, for example, or to a white woman, or someone with a disability. The way different aspects of our identities intersect will impact how we are perceived (either consciously or unconsciously) by those around us. I like to think of intersectionality as the crossroads between racialised identity, status, lived experiences and gender identity. In yoga these comprise the mental and physical connection, and mental and physical practices.

Yoga classes for different identities

In a perfect world I would like to think that all identities would feel comfortable to attend any class – but unfortunately that is not the current reality, although this is changing. I believe that there is still a need to have classes that cater for different identities, because it allows an environment to be created where everyone can feel comfortable without the fear of being judged or receiving unnecessary attention, somewhere they will feel accepted and be with people they can identify with. There is a plethora of reasons for the need, all of which reinforce the purpose behind why I created Curvesomeyoga. Some people will prefer 'plus-size classes', 'women-only classes' and 'Black, indigenous and people of colour (BIPOC) classes'. I think that all people are ultimately looking for are judgement-free spaces, and feel that they will only get this with people who look like them. For instance, I have taught women-only classes because there is a real need for this; the women have stated that they have felt safer and confident in these types of classes. In an ideal world everyone would feel safe and comfortable to attend any class, but for now separate classes are much needed, as they give people the opportunity to experience yoga.

Recent initiatives to offer yoga classes and retreats exclusively for Black women or other marginalised groups show how times have changed, and although they can still attract negative comments, there is greater acknowledgement that these types of classes are needed. The fact that I could co-create a festival for the Black community during 2020 in the middle of the pandemic serves to confirm this. The feedback has been excellent, indicating that there is indeed a need for events that create a safe, judgement-free space where communities can have access to teachers who can understand their experiences and there is less chance of trauma being triggered. That is not to say that I don't still get negative feedback – I recall advertising a body positive yoga class for people who were a UK size 14 or over and was accused of discrimination. However, I believe we must get over our thoughts about division and create what is needed to allow everyone to access yoga.

It all comes back to understanding that the dominant group (i.e. those with power, who are normally white) wants us all to achieve the perceived 'ideal body'. As we know, diets don't always work – but it's an industry that is worth billions every year. Instead, we should celebrate our differences and uniqueness. Why should we have to adhere to these very limiting criteria when we are so much more? How we choose to personally identify ourselves should be completely down to individual choice rather than being a square peg trying to fit into a round hole. As we know, identity can be a very delicate subject, and we are not always in agreement with the ways in which society endeavours to label us. This feeling of not fitting in or being accepted for who we truly are can account for a lot of the anxiety and stress that we see in society nowadays; people don't feel they can claim their true identity for fear of being different and the consequences that may follow.

Trauma

Although we construct our identities to some extent, society does too. Our identities are an important part of us as they affect the way we interact with the world and how society interacts with us. Unfortunately, these interactions are not always pleasant and can lead to trauma. For instance, the Black community face daily racial micro- and macroaggressions, which can affect people both physically and mentally. There has always been evidence of this, but it's now being more widely reported and shared on social media. The rise of the Black Lives Matter movement is a clear example of heightened awareness around racial discrimination due to social media.

Trauma can be experienced in a number of ways, and can have

a huge impact on the individuals and communities experiencing it. Not all signs of stress are visible. For example, according to biographer Taylor Branch (1968), Martin Luther King's autopsy revealed that, though only 39 years old, he 'had the heart of a 60 year old'. Branch attributed this to the stress of 13 years in the civil rights movement – it had literally aged his heart.

The premise of historical trauma theory (a relatively new concept in public health) is that populations historically subjected to long-term mass trauma (colonialism, slavery, war, genocide, etc.) exhibit a higher prevalence of disease even several generations after the original trauma occurred. I have gained a greater understanding of this from reading Dr Gail Parker's book, *Restorative Yoga for Ethnic and Race-Based Stress and Trauma* (2020). The book outlines and explains how trauma, stress and PTSD can be passed down to future generations. It is a must-read book that gives great insight and examples of the traumas encountered based on race. We must not forget that segregation in the US was still in place not that long ago – in 1964 Black people were still not welcome in specific spaces. In South Africa, apartheid was law until the 1990s. This is mind-blowing!

I am so glad to see that historical trauma is now being acknowledged and discussed more widely within the wellness space, particularly in trauma-based yoga. That is why I think it would be an excellent idea for trauma-based yoga to be incorporated within all teacher training courses to provide teachers with a fundamental understanding of some of the issues students may bring into the yoga space. As teachers, we don't have a crystal ball, so being armed with the appropriate training(s) and knowledge is the next best thing. Earlier this year I completed Mei Lai Swan's Yoga for Humankind Trauma-Informed Yoga and Embodied Social Change training course (https://yogafor humankind.org) and cannot recommend it highly enough. The training covered so many topics that I had found to be missing in many of the trainings I attended at the start of my yoga journey, and it gave me a lot to think about. For example, the silence and stillness that we endeavour to cultivate within a yoga space may be overwhelming and trigger traumatic memories for some; for example, asking students not to move might bring back a memory of not having the ability to move.

In order to avoid this we need to give the students permission to come out of the pose whenever they wish. This serves to demonstrate that we cannot know what kind of trauma a student might be (consciously or unconsciously) holding when they attend one of our classes.

Yoga is often a form of refuge or safe space and a space of healing from daily experiences, but, unfortunately, it can also sometimes be a space that creates trauma through a teacher's implicit biases. This can be seen where stereotypes are perpetuated – for instance, where it is assumed that anyone in an abundant body is likely to be unhealthy or if judgements are made about someone's practice based on their size or on their appearance. Teachers want to make their yoga spaces more diverse, but one of the fundamental problems is the lack of understanding of the barriers and challenges that the local community face daily. Here are some questions to consider:

- Do marginalised communities see themselves when they enter yoga spaces?
- Do you have the knowledge and expertise to teach to diverse communities so that you have an appreciation and under-standing of the barriers the community face when they enter your space?
- What steps are you taking to dismantle white supremacy? Is it enough just to claim inclusivity?
- Do you take yoga off the mat and champion for social justice (ahimsa)?

These questions may make you feel uncomfortable, but they are important. Just as I have learnt how to question my initial assump-tions about yoga's roots, we must all keep striving to be self-aware, learning more about our own biases and what we have learnt in the past. Like yoga, the world around us is constantly evolving!

6

Appropriate Language

*We tend to look through language and not real-
ise how much power language has.*

Deborah Tannen, author

Our body image is affected by the words that we use and that others use about us. Before we look at terminology, we need to really question whether it's our business to label a body or define it with our own categorisations. Many such definitions stem from current metrics (e.g. body mass index, or BMI), but are these really fit for purpose? We also need to be aware that some of the words that describe bodies can be used as weapons to deliberately harm.

Terminology

The best approach, especially for teachers, is to ask people how they would like to be referred to – this goes for body type and for gender identity. It's also a good idea to acknowledge that what an individual wants to be called or how they want to talk about their experiences is up to them and should not be defined by us.

Altering the language we use to talk about weight can reduce stigma. While many people are uncomfortable with certain terms, others may choose to use them. This can be seen as an act of rebellion or a way to neutralise a word that has previously been wielded against them – or they may simply feel that it's the most appropriate word to describe their body. Below are some examples.

Overweight

The term 'overweight' implies that there is a natural weight that people should be and that everyone should have the same proportions of height and weight. However, BMI is inaccurate as it does not take into account muscle mass, bone density, body shape, racialised identity or gender.

The standard weight status categories associated with BMI ranges for adults internationally are:

- A BMI of 18.49 or below means a person is underweight.
- A BMI of 18.5 to 24.99 means they are of normal weight.
- A BMI of 25 to 29.99 means they are overweight.
- A BMI of 30 or above is supposed to indicate that a person is ob*se.

Fat

Unlike most descriptors, the word 'fat' isn't always considered neutral. It's often framed in negativity and can be used to cause emotional harm and insult. That's why I can understand why some people find the use of the word 'fat' traumatic and triggering. However, some individuals have reclaimed the word and use it solely as an objective description. Using the word neutrally removes any negative associations and therefore doesn't allow it to be used as an insult.

Interestingly, back in the late 1300s, the word 'fat' had several positive meanings, including 'fertile' and 'abundant', and in the 1600s it had an underlying sense of prosperity (e.g. the phrase 'fat cat' to describe wealth or affluence).

Fat phobia is seen as an inherently overt type of discrimination – calling people horrible names relating to their weight, bullying them because of their weight, and so on – but it's a lot more nuanced than that. Health is also often used as a subtle and sometimes non-subtle way of shaming somebody about their weight (e.g. the phrase 'a moment on the lips, a lifetime on the hips'). The medical industry also often assumes that a curvy person's health concerns must be related to their weight, when often this is not the case, and fails to take their issues seriously.

Curvy

'Curvy' has fewer negative connotations than 'fat' – and this is why I chose the word 'curve' to be part of Curvesomeyoga. But there are some individuals who take issue with it, because not all women above a size UK 12 are considered curvy. I like that it's a term that isn't used to offend or cause harm.

Ob*se

The word 'ob*se' is a medical term that has so many negative connotations. It's a word that I try not to use as I have personally witnessed how triggering it can be when used as clickbait or to sensationalise conversations. The word is usually viewed as undesirable and its use often offends and can cause distress.

Plus size

The retailer Lane Bryant coined the term 'plus' in advertisements for 'Misses Plus Size'. It continues to be the most common way to refer to clothing in UK size 14 and up in the retail industry. The 'plus' refers to being outside 'standard' sizing. Some individuals are fighting to eradicate the use of this term.

Straight size

'Straight size' is another fashion industry term, used for clothing sizes not termed 'plus size', or the size most designers use as a model. It also appears to be adopted as part of eating disorder professionals' language in an attempt to be more inclusive.

Skinny

Skinny can be considered similar to 'thin', a term I consider to be neutral, but in a way that can be considered unattractive, and implies being unhealthy or even underweight. I don't like the term 'skinny' for this very reason and personally prefer the term 'slim', as for me it is neutral. If you have to use the term 'skinny' do so carefully, as some people may find being described as skinny offensive.

Disability

A disability is 'a physical or mental impairment that has a "substantial" and "long-term" negative effect on your ability to do normal daily activities' (Equality Act 2010). This definition replaces the similar provisions in the Disability Discrimination Act 1995. The definition of disability does not only refer to people who are visibly disabled, for example those who are blind, or have mobility difficulties, like wheelchair users. It also includes a broad range of conditions like depression, diabetes, dyslexia, dyspraxia, autism, cancer, multiple sclerosis and schizophrenia.

The terminology has changed over the years and we are seeing different terms that are considered more neutral, as the term has some negative connotations. It should be noted that people with disabilities are *people*, and I would advise that you refer to the person first followed by the disability. For example, Elaine Hughes suggests that one should say, 'My friend has autism and may not understand social questions', rather than 'My autistic friend may not understand social questions.' As always, it is best to ask the person how they wish to be identified.

At present there are various terms relating to disability, and current literature encourages people to focus on the person's ability. So you hear words such as 'differently abled', 'person with a disability' or 'disabled'. Some countries are actively encouraging people to drop the term 'disabled' in favour of 'differently abled', stating that 'disabled' is now a negative word. As a disabled person born with a physical disability, I take no offence at the term 'disabled', and this word is recognised by the UN. I recognise my disability and I view it as a true reflection of what I can and cannot do. I am disabled from doing certain tasks and, yes, I may find alternative ways to do what I need to do. However, I believe the word is a true reflection of my disability. I have no issue with people referring to me as a disabled person or a person with a disability. I would suggest speaking to the individual about how they want to be referred to.

Elaine Hughes, Disability Champion and consultant

Pronouns

A pronoun is a word that refers either to the person talking (I, me), the person they are talking to (you), or someone or something that is being talked about (she, it, them, this). Gender pronouns (she/he/they) are used to refer to people, and relate to someone's personal sense of their own identity and how they choose to express their gender, perhaps in their physical appearance. When we are talking about individuals, we refer to them as:

- she/her/hers
- he/him/his
- they/them, or any other preferred pronouns.

Never assume someone's gender based on the way that they look or dress, as it may not represent their gender identity. It should also be noted that not all individuals will identify as a particular gender, and that is the beauty of diversity – the freedom to be and express yourself as you wish. For further information on gender identity and pronouns, see www.mypronouns.org/how and https://uwm.edu/lgbtrc/support/gender-pronouns.

The importance of language

The words we use carry certain connotations and emotions. We should pick them carefully because they can define us and create a lasting impression. The words we speak carry so much fragility and yet so much weight. They form one of the fundamental ways in which we communicate and reveal so much about who we are and what we stand for. Since the dawn of time, words have provided us with a way to form connection or division. There are so many paradoxes with language, and people may understand words differently depending on societal factors. We can also unintentionally reveal things about ourselves through our words.

Using more inclusive language

As yoga teachers, we must be open to reflecting on ways to be more inclusive and understand that our choice of language is critically important. Our words have the power to inspire and heal, or devastate, traumatise, cause harm or make students feel they don't belong. I disagree with the adage 'sticks and stones...' – words can harm us, especially trying to create an environment that lacks judgement.

We can all feel vulnerable on the yoga mat; it's a place where we open ourselves up to let things go, which may bring up emotions and long-held feelings. Students may feel open to criticism because their body doesn't conform to what is classed as a 'yoga body'. Language is one of the most complete ways in which we can discriminate. By using inclusive and adaptive language, everybody is allowed to benefit from the practice, rather than only a few. Our words really influence the yoga space – we therefore need to take care when establishing our vocabulary in order to create a safe space for everyone. Feeling excluded can certainly cause students to lose a sense of safety.

Teachers can teach the same style of yoga class but elicit different responses; through the choice of words, students can feel empowered or disempowered. This resonates with me, having practised numerous hot yoga classes where the dialogue was the same, but the experience completely different in terms of the energy and the focus of the class.

Self-study is an important way in which we can become aware of the language that we use so that we can avoid causing unintentional harm. As we have seen, language is a key component in allowing our students to feel safe, and this includes the way we identify them and refer to them. One thing we certainly want to avoid is our students feeling 'othered' (see the section 'Othering' below).

History shows us that language, communication and experiences continually evolve. This means we can rewrite the proverbial script and create vocabularies that are more compassionate and inclusive – vocabularies that allow everyone to feel welcome. Language isn't meant to alienate us; it's meant to help us understand one another and create connection.

Some dos and don'ts

Language is very deeply ingrained, and therein lies the problem. Our vocabulary reflects our cultures, families, friends, identity and community. We need to become aware of our own biases – often picked up from people we have met, the media we've consumed throughout our lives, and our lived experiences. How do we begin to address this? The answer is through education and training.

Listening more and speaking less is a great way to be aware of our biases and what we tend to say. Nowadays, we live busy lives and are often on autopilot; 'Think before we speak' should be our mantra, as most words flow out before our brains even engage.

'Just'

How many times have you used the word 'just' in your teaching? It might seem like a simple throwaway word that seems to effortlessly fit into our vocabulary and appears to have no real meaning, but it has so many negative connotations. Have you ever considered the impact that this word has on someone? Chances are, you've used phrases similar to 'Just put your right foot between your hands' or Nike's famous slogan 'Just do it'. Its use is actually considered to be ableist and can instantly snap someone out of their mindful yoga practice.

I've started to have this conversation about 'just' frequently. Originally I didn't accept the frequency with which I used it. I was so wrong – no one was more surprised than me when I listened to a recording of myself where I cued the entry into a posture with 'just'. I put myself in my students' shoes and thought about how I'd feel if a teacher said, 'Just go into splits' – I'd feel inadequate, because the use of 'just' makes it sound like something that should be achieved effortlessly, and I know that the rest of the class would not be a nice experience. I'm currently considering creating a 'just' jar – like a traditional swear jar, but for 'justs'.

Listening to one of my own recorded classes was an excellent way to experience my use of language. It made me aware of the words that I use as fillers as well as their frequency. I seem to love describing everything as 'good' or 'perfect', and this is something I'm consciously working to remove, particularly in the context of when I'm asking anyone to do something in class. Using praise in this way is unhelpful as it contradicts me telling my students that there is no such thing as yoga perfect, that it is a practice, or that falling out of the pose is okay as this is all part of being yogi. As no one is perfect, perfection should have no place on the yoga mat. The use of ableist language doesn't make you a bad person; I've found that its use is often unintentional. Avoid generalising and create a space that is inclusive.

Guys

Assume that you don't know anything about how people identify in class but take the opportunity to welcome everyone. One of the generalisations that needs to be avoided is referring to large groups as 'guys'. What's wrong with saying, 'Hi guys', you might ask. It's seen by many as a ubiquitous term used to address any gender and is hence considered gender-neutral – but is harmful. It's a phrase that I used regularly, but I am making a conscious effort to stop using it. It's funny how we absorb things vicariously, including words, especially when you hear them used so regularly that they become ingrained.

So, let's break it down; at first glance, 'guys' seems inviting and friendly, but it undoubtedly has masculine connotations. Although used as a default term in Western societies, it probably shouldn't be normalised as an all-encompassing phrase. The term may be commonly used, but from an inclusive perspective it may be considered inconsiderate to subconsciously address only one specific gender. It could also be difficult for women or gender non-conforming people to feel empowered when, upon receiving a greeting, they're immediately misgendered or ignored.

It may initially be difficult to remove a word or phrase from your vocabulary, but being conscious of potential negative implications and starting to erase their use is a good place to start. In the case of 'guys', once I have found an alternative term that I am comfortable using to refer to a specific group of individuals, this will become easier. Some alternative ways in which you can greet the class are 'friends', 'everyone', 'humans', 'folks' or 'beautiful people'. I remember when I was teaching in Texas a teacher called Brad would try to get me to say 'ya'll' – but not with much success (the memory still makes me smile).

Do not openly refer to students' genders, as you do not know how the people in the room wish to be identified. The only instance where this will be appropriate is if you are able to find out everyone's pronouns before the beginning of class. One way I try to work around this is addressing the students by their names; I feel that it is so much more personal. How do you feel when someone acknowledges you by your name? – It's so lovely to be seen. However, it's been suggested that it is a good idea to get permission to use someone's name, as some students may not want to draw attention to themselves in the class, so bear this in mind.

Non-gendered language

I love these examples provided by Susanna Barkataki.

- Replace 'pregnant women' with 'pregnant people'.
- Instead of saying 'menstruating ladies' replace with 'anyone menstruating'.

Describing body types in a pose

By creating body diversity within classes we begin to see the unique-ness of bodies and honour them. Consider moving away from using body parts or clothing as reference points, as these can prove to be confusing for students and can also be gendered; for instance, telling people to place their hands in line with their bra strap. Instead of these landmarks, use other reference points as alignment cues – the mat (long or short side) or places in the room (front of the room or ceiling), or specific measurements (three feet distance apart). We often cue the feet to be hip distance apart, but students may not be aware of this measurement. I like to say, 'place your feet to whatever distance feels comfortable', or alternatively 'have the feet at least two fists' distance apart' (which can be demonstrated) to help with awareness. I've found that using these alternatives eliminates some of the confused expressions that I used to see in class.

Another example of gender bias is when I've heard teachers say, 'Men may find Chaturanga easier as they have greater upper body strength.' Although this may be true for some men, we can't assume this to be the case for everyone, and there are plenty of women who are able to do Chaturanga (four-limbed staff pose) with ease. This kind of phrasing is unhelpful and may make students feel uncom-fortable. An alternative, to make this statement less gendered, is 'You may find Chaturanga easier if you tend to have more strength in your upper body.'

Take steps to decolonise your classes

Where possible, we have to work towards decolonising our classes. One way to do so is by understanding exactly what we are saying. For instance, I no longer chant in my classes, for a number of rea-sons. I would never chant 'Jesus, Jesus' in a class, as someone could find that offensive, but that may be equivalent to what we are doing when we are asked to chant. Sometimes, we don't know why or what we are chanting but we repeat it verbatim because this is what we were taught during teacher training. In doing so, we may be causing harm to someone for whom yoga is part of their heritage and who is offended by how yoga is being appropriated. If you do decide to chant, make sure that you understand the meaning and explain it to the students. It's also important to ensure that they are aware that taking part in chanting is not mandatory.

Saying 'Namaste' has become the default way to close a class, but this needs to be examined. I'm aware that not saying 'Namaste' can cause confusion among students as it has become a common signifier of the end of a class. Literally practised and translated, it means 'bow to you' and is a greeting of respect (Barkataki, 2020), but some students may become offended as the term is often used incorrectly. Instead, there are a number of alternative ways to end class – 'thank you', 'go in peace', 'from my heart to yours', 'thank you for practising with me' or 'giving gratitude'. I believe the point is not that you cannot end the class with 'Namaste', but that you need to know and understand the context in which it is appropriate to use it. If you would like to find out more, check out Susanna Barkataki's website for a downloadable PDF that explains some alternative ways to end your class (www.susannabarkataki.com/post/namaste), or check out her book *Embrace Yoga's Roots* (Barkataki, 2020).

Othering

Othering is a phenomenon in which some individuals or groups are defined and labelled as not fitting in within the norms of a social group. It also involves attributing negative characteristics to people or groups that differentiate them from the perceived normative social group (Cherry, 2020). Othering Black people in wellness spaces takes away the safety of these spaces and serves to maintain the white wellness status quo that has long been prevalent.

This occurs is in statements like:

- I wish I had a booty like yours!
- I am the same colour as you are now.

I've heard these examples a lot, and they are not unique to the wellness space. The latter usually occurs when someone returns from a holiday and wants to highlight their tan. I often wonder how this can ever be seen as an innocent statement or how it's supposed to create a greater connection – if this is how you connect, you need to think about the type of connection you are endeavouring to create. Likewise, using stereotypes (such as the booty) is not the best way to try to connect with Black students, and this practice must be stopped. Anything that causes a student not to have the best experience possible in a class must be removed.

If you are a teacher and witness something akin to this, you need to call it out – even if you are not the one perpetuating this practice. I'm so glad that we are starting to live in a world where we are becoming more respectful and aware of the implications of our language and behaviour, and being held more accountable for our actions. If this change can happen within a yoga space, and taken off the mat too, imagine how much better the world will be.

Never judge a yogi by their looks

We cannot look at someone and be able to assess their ability. Individuals should not be judged by their shape, size, age or ethnicity, or be measured against what is thought of as a 'yogi body', before they get on the mat.

> During my teacher training I felt the teacher didn't always understand why I couldn't do certain binds. Sometimes people seem surprised that a larger person can be as flexible as I am. I have had people be surprised to find out I was the teacher of the class, rather than a student.
>
> *Saskia Bolscher, yoga teacher*

Assumptions of ability should not be based on looks. However, this seems to be very much what is happening in many yoga spaces, and it is wrong on so many levels. Creating language that supports the experience that you are trying to offer to your students is a powerful instrument for any teacher.

> *Words cast spells, that's why it's called SPELLING. Words are energy. Use them wisely!*

Source unknown

7

Marketing Yourself as a Body Positive Yoga Teacher

*Diversity is being invited to the party, and
inclusion is being asked to dance.®*

Verná Myers, The Verná Myers Company

I love this quote so much that I've adapted it for a yoga context:

**Diversity is being invited to yoga, equality is being able to access
yoga and inclusion is being allowed to practice.**

The teacher's role is ever evolving, just like the great practice of yoga.
Yoga teachers have now become part of the media by virtue of having
to promote yoga in the form of advertising, blogging, writing, and
so on. Although all this provides us with different ways in which to
engage potential students, sometimes I miss the days where all I had
to think about was teaching.

Marketing and publicity are now a part of allowing yoga to be
truly accessible and inclusive so that potential students, regardless of
their background or ability, will feel welcome at class before they even
step onto the yoga mat. Many potential students may be reluctant to
get started because they don't feel they belong. This stems from the
fact that they are not visible in mainstream marketing campaigns.
Although this is starting to change, there is still a long way to go.

FIERCE GRACE: AN EXAMPLE OF DIVERSE MARKETING

One of the first UK yoga studios that went against conventional marketing norms was Fierce Grace, the brainchild of Michele Pernetta. The publicity campaign they created was pioneering and radical, and fully embraced the ethos of showing regular bodies doing yoga, people you would not usually see in mainstream advertising. It was ahead of its time in the London yoga scene and really stood out for me as the images used reflected the studios' community.

The campaign worked. When attending classes at Fierce Grace studios you could see a diverse range of people of different abilities and backgrounds practising yoga.

Marketing and publicity

Most teachers will find that marketing is an important part of their business (it's not essential, but it helps). I certainly found this when I set up Curvesomeyoga and started offering body positive classes outside of the studio environment.

Who do you want to serve?

First, you need to decide which community you wish to serve – this may be considered finding your niche. I suggest going back to why you want to teach yoga and what you wish to achieve. For example, I created Curvesomeyoga because I wanted to offer classes for anyone who did not feel welcome within mainstream yoga classes or those who didn't see people like them represented in the advertising. This resulted in me offering classes targeted at the body positive community. You need to know your audience and have a client avatar in mind when you start to market your classes. This is so that you don't do what I call 'spray and pray' marketing, meaning that you advertise everywhere (Facebook, Twitter, Instagram, etc.) and pray that you will reach your client. Knowing your target audience allows you to speak directly to your ideal clients.

The power of language

Make your class descriptions clear – potential students won't necessarily know Hatha from Vinyasa. There's so much choice out there and it's our job to help them make the right choice as easily as possible. Always go back to the beginner's mind – this will help you to strike the right balance in terms of what information you provide. What do you wish you had known before getting on the mat? It's better to have too much information than too little. This is also your opportunity to make students aware of any practices that are included in the experience – hands-on adjustments, the use of oils or music, whether it is a chair-based class, and so on. This removes any element of surprise and provides students with the ability to make informed choices. Providing information will evoke feelings of safety for your students and eliminate any anxiety or fears they may have, allowing them to have the best experience possible in your class. This, in turn, will make them want to come back time and time again. Allow students and potential students to contact you regarding any questions or concerns they have, especially beginners. This is also an opportunity for potential students to find out a little bit about you as a teacher.

We need to be intentional in how we welcome different body types. I learnt that the more specific I made my marketing descriptions, the more successful I was in reaching this audience. I would state 'absolutely no experience required' or 'classes for size 12 or above' so that there was no room for confusion and students knew exactly what they were signing up for. For mixed classes I was sure to explain that everyone was welcome, regardless of shape, size, gender, ethnicity or ability. I would also create polls to understand the types of classes future students wanted and then market these accordingly. Remember, a body positive class does not have to be a particular style of yoga (you could teach a Hatha yoga or a Vinyasa flow class with the body positive principles in mind, for example), so it's important to ensure that your classes are described clearly.

Recently I wondered why there was still an absence of certain body types in the yoga space – even in classes marketed as being accessible – when there's evidence on so many body positive platforms that there's an interest in yoga. I found out that the language used in the marketing was the issue. The word 'inclusive' was not sufficient; I had to stipulate that it was a plus-size yoga class to ensure that potential students would feel safe enough to participate.

Make yourself visible

Students want to know about you and this in turn will allow them to feel welcome at your classes. You are your energy and students need to see you. This means being visible on your social media channels, and this is a great way for you to show up authentically. You can start by showing behind-the-scenes elements of your daily life – for example, you going for a walk and sharing your environment and talking about it. I did this for a long time before getting in front of the camera. When I started promoting body positive classes I made a conscious decision not use any images of myself. However, years later I was made to realise the importance of making myself more visible, so that I could be part of the representation that was missing from yoga.

Imagery

The way in which we use content to publicise yoga classes can be very powerful in either welcoming or excluding students. We need to consider how our content may unintentionally create a barrier to the practice of yoga.

As well as showing yourself in your marketing, consider what other types of imagery you're sharing – does it reflect ableism, that is, do the images show poses that will not be achievable for the majority of potential students? How often do you see images of yogis in poses such as Savasana or Sukhasana (easy pose)? Are these considered boring or not aesthetically pleasing? Yoga is not all about looks, it's about the feelings – but can we demonstrate how yoga makes us feel? Can you think of an alternative way to demonstrate yoga instead of using asana?

There are many people who wish to do yoga but are scared by stereotypical images that don't reflect them. An image paints a thousand words; it can be welcoming or exclusionary. It would seem that some parts of the yoga industry have chosen the lens of the popular magazine to sell yoga. You could be forgiven for mixing up a yoga magazine cover with that of a mainstream women's magazine. This was pointed out to me during December 2020 when the cover of one yoga magazine showed a young, slim, white yogi in a red bikini in Vrksasana. Images like this just add to distorting yoga's image and associating it with fitness.

Tara's experience provides us with an example of publicity leading to stereotypes:

> I've always loved the idea of yoga: spending an hour on the mat and forgetting about the stresses of daily life. Despite only ever seeing skinny women who look great in leggings and a crop top doing yoga, I didn't let those stereotypes put me off trying it. I think that any kind of fitness should be open to everyone.

When I created Curvesomeyoga I became very intentional about the images and language that I used to show that yoga had no size. Representation really matters – how can students be what they can't see? I wanted people to become curious enough about yoga so that they could experience its benefits, so I used images of diverse yogis sharing their yoga practice and disrupting the yoga space – Dianne Bondy, Jessamyn Stanley and Dana Falsetti. The issue was that these yogis were all American, and I could not find any yogis from the UK to challenge the limited yoga body rhetoric.

In my marketing, I created ads that specifically show diverse bodies. I also decided to go one step further and collaborated with some members of the body positive community and created a yoga video (available at https://youtu.be/XFxfuOo_BkU). To date it has had over

195,800 views! The purpose was to show curvy yogis practising yoga. I even had meetings and conversations with actor Lisa Riley and TV presenter Alison Hammond about supporting Curvesomeyoga. The reaction to the video and images demonstrated how marketing and imagery have the ability to create positive change and provided me with the back-up I needed to encourage people onto the mat.

Creating short videos of my yoga classes (with permission from the students) has provided me with a great way to demonstrate that yoga is everyone's birthright. These videos are nothing fancy. I use the time-lapse option on my phone to show a short Surya Namaskar (sun salutation) sequence and share it on social media. Such videos have resulted in new students enquiring about yoga.

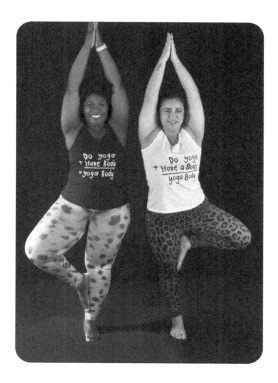

I've found that education, demystifying yoga and sharing its benefits is the best way to successfully change people's perceptions and reassure them that yoga is indeed for them.

8

Using Props

You can entice a yogi to the mat, but you cannot force them to use props.

I'm pleased to see that using props during yoga asana practice is becoming more popular, as they're a great way to make yoga postures more accessible for everyone by providing support, creating length and helping with alignment. They can also aid rehabilitation following injury by providing support, as well as being excellent tools for strength building and creating balance. For all these reasons, their use should be core to any yoga class.

There still seems to be some stigma attached to the use of props. For instance, those using them may be made to feel that they are less capable, that props are only for beginners, or that using props slows the class down. There are even myths that real yogis do not use props. All of this results in a reluctance to use them. However, there are many benefits to using props and, when used in certain ways, they can actually make the practice more challenging.

Normalising the use of props will help to encourage their use. One way to remove stigma around using props is to set up the class with the relevant props in situ for everyone so that no one feels singled out; you could also use the props yourself when demonstrating poses. Allow the chosen prop to be part of the pose rather than offered as an option. As teachers, we normalise the use of props very simply by using them ourselves, and you will invariably find that students will copy you. However, this can take time, so don't be put off and stay with it. For instance, after attending Accessible

Yoga training, I was all fired up, and the first opportunity I got I sat at the front of the class in a chair and invited the class to join me. Only one student took me up on the offer, so we started the Surya Namaskar sequence in the chair while the remainder of the class did the mat-based variation. However, on another occasion (in a local church hall where the students were more representative of the local community) most students joined me in doing a chair-based practice, swapping between the chair and the mat as the class progressed. It was so wonderful to witness the future of yoga – everyone had agency over their practice and did their own version of the yoga postures. There was never any doubt in my mind that this was possible, but I'd like for this to be the norm, not the exception.

When teaching online, remember that not everyone will have yoga props to hand. Encourage students to be creative and use household items as alternatives if they do not have the recommended items to hand. The most common yoga props are described in the following section, with some suggestions for alternatives.

Types of props
Yoga mat
Although ubiquitous, mats are not necessarily essential. Many of us may not be aware that we are using a yoga mat as a prop: it provides us with stability so that we do not slip, in addition to providing padding and cushioning to help to protect the body and joints. Mats can also be rolled up to create other props (i.e. bolsters).

Some alternatives to yoga mats are carpet, a woven blanket, grippy socks, a bed or wooden flooring.

Yoga blocks and bricks
These are perhaps the most used props. As well as supporting the yoga practice, they can also make it more challenging. Blocks and bricks can help bring the floor closer to the student and are also good for strength building. The body sometimes likes to go with the path of least resistance, so the provision of support is welcome in helping

to maintain an element of alignment. For instance, in Trikonasana (triangle pose), using a block permits the arm to lengthen towards the floor while not losing the shape of the posture. Another common use for blocks is to sit on them to allow the hips to be higher than the knees, assisting with the opening of the hips. I use my blocks for this on a regular basis.

Blocks can also be used to help engage particular muscles. For example, a block can be placed between the inner thighs during Setu Bandhasana (bridge pose). They can also allow students to hold postures for a longer duration, for instance by placing one beneath the sacrum in supported Setu Bandhasana.

Blocks come in various sizes, but I always recommend my students use larger cork blocks as these are sturdy and allow the students to feel secure. The height of the blocks can be adjusted to accommodate individual bodies, and it's worth reminding students of this during class.

Alternatives to blocks include firm cushions, folded blankets or a stack of large books.

Yoga straps/belts

Yoga straps and belts can help to find the ease in the pose, eliminate resistance and maintain alignment. This can be seen when providing support in restorative poses such as Supta Baddha Konasana (reclined cobbler's pose), where a looped belt can be placed around the waist and the outside of the feet in order to support the legs.

A strap can also be used to create length in the arms, allowing the student to release tension when over-stretching may occur. For instance, looping a strap around the feet in Paschimottanasana (seated forward bend) creates length in the arms, especially when students are not comfortable when reaching for the feet, helping with the alignment of the shoulders and bringing a sense of ease to the pose. It can also be useful in postures where the hands meet (e.g. Gomukasana (cow face pose)) or during binds. Using the straps to bind the arms and legs to help achieve alignment, for example in Chaturanga where the arms tend to splay out, can also make the posture more challenging.

The yoga belt can help in any positions that cause the students to feel as though they are being suffocated by their breasts. This tends to occur in Salamba Sarvangasana and Adho Mukha Svanasana (downward-facing dog) for yogis who are abundant in this area of the body. The belt is wrapped around the upper chest (high on the breast line, or just at the breast tissue pectoral area), and is then tightened to help to prevent the breasts sliding down.

A yoga strap can be replaced with a necktie, scarf, bathrobe belt, sock or towel. If buckling is required, a cloth belt with a loop closure will suffice.

Bolsters

Bolsters can provide connection to the ground in poses like Balasana or literally provide support as students relax and let go in Savasana when placed under the knees, or in Supta Baddha Konasana when placed beneath the thighs.

A good alternative to a bolster is pillows that are bound together, or folded blankets.

Chair

We are starting to see an increase in the number of chair yoga classes being offered, which is great. The fact that it can be done by everyone, and even at a student's desk in the office, means that if students are injured they can continue their practice. Chair yoga is also another way to make yoga accessible for everyone – if the teacher has the ability to teach both chair and mat-based yoga simultaneously, they can create a mixed-level class.

The book *Accessible Yoga* by Jivana Heyman (2019) is a good resource that shares the chair variations of poses. A chair is an awesome prop for students who have less mobility and prefer to do a seated practice. It can also provide support by raising the floor or providing a base to perform balances (e.g. Surya Namaskar or plank poses). I recommend that students use the chair if they don't have confidence or have difficulty getting down and up from the floor. You may find that yoga is the first time where they attempt this – and after a time the chair may become redundant. While the chair is supporting the weight of the body it provides stability but also allows the students to extend legs in standing poses, for example. I have had students share with me that they would deliberately avoid sitting on the floor in social settings for fear of not being able to get up again. I am happy to say that this changed once they got the confidence to do so after practising yoga.

Ensure that the chair does not have wheels, to eliminate the risk of it sliding, and place it on the mat. Ideally you could use a yoga chair, which is a modified version of a standard metal chair. You can find a range of yoga chairs at Yogamatters (see www.yogamatters.com/collections/yoga-chairs-feet-up).

Alternatives to chairs include coffee tables, sofas and beds.

Wall

I fondly refer to the wall as 'Paul the wall'. Providing wall-based variations allows the orientation of a pose to be changed if necessary, and can be especially useful if floor-based poses are challenging (e.g. Bakasana or Adho Mukha Svanasana). The same applies for balancing postures. Vrksasana and Garudasana (eagle pose) are good examples as they can be done with the back against the wall to provide stability.

The wall is also great for helping students to feel how a posture should be aligned. I often say that 'the body will always try to be lazy and go the way of least resistance'. For example, in Vrksasana the student may place the foot on the thigh, but in order to keep the foot in place they may allow the butt to stick out rather than pushing the pelvis forward. Taking the pose to the wall is a good way to help them become aware of this habit or action. Once they have this awareness, they will start to place the foot below the knee to maintain alignment and, in the meantime, as the body opens accordingly, they are building the foundations of the pose. I will then ask them to come back to the mat and see if this has helped them to better understand what they were trying to achieve; they also have the option to stay at the wall.

Yoga wheel

The yoga wheel is a hollow, cylinder-shaped prop designed to aid stretching, release tension and improve flexibility. It's very versatile! The wheel can be used to make postures more relaxing by providing support – for instance, placing the wheel underneath the sacrum for supported Setu Bandhasana.

The yoga wheel has become one of my favourite props. It allows me to be so creative with my yoga practice, challenging me and providing ease at the same time. You can find me balancing on it or simply draped over it, just relaxing and enjoying the deep stretch that I'm being afforded.

I ran a workshop on using the yoga wheel, and someone who had a frozen shoulder was able to use it to help work towards recovery. Being able to access a pose in a way that had not previously been possible gave her hope.

I am wheely a wheel girl at heart now. Apologies for the poor attempt at humour, but I could not resist! I promise I will stick to the day job.

Debunking myths about props
'Real yogis never used props'

Some teachers or schools of yoga discourage the use of props based on the idea that props were not a part of the early practitioners' practice. On the contrary, it would seem that the use of props is not such a modern phenomenon of yoga as some believe. The use of a cloth yoga strap or belt (yogapatta) to fix one's body in a posture is at least 2000 years old – almost as old as yoga itself. The straps were used to help yogis who were in seated postures for long periods of time.

The body has been considered the first and original prop:

> For me, prop is not only for the asana. It should contribute to the position of the body which in turn can let the mind be calm and state of 'chitta vritti nirodha' be experienced. Body is my first prop. The body is a prop to the soul [sic]. (B. K. S. Iyengar, cited in Powell, 2018)

It appears that props did not have a linear evolution before being reintroduced to modern-day yoga by B. K. S. Iyengar, who used them to accommodate his personal practice. He introduced the use of the buckle on the yoga strap, as well as the various ways in which it can be used to enhance postures.

The floor is a fundamental prop in yoga, and might be one of the most overlooked. We use it to ground ourselves and to help us to find balance. So, from the outset we are all invariably incorporating props. In a body positive class, using the floor is a great way to change the orientation of the pose in order to make it more accessible.

'More experienced students never use props'

There are some perceptions that props are a bad thing and are only used by less experienced students, especially when in mixed-level classes. In these situations, the use of props may make some students feel inferior; they will see students doing poses without props and may feel this is somehow 'better' or desirable. However, it's important to emphasise that props can aid the yoga practice in numerous ways; in the words of Dianne Bondy, they can make postures feel more luxurious. One way in which I try to challenge the perception that experienced students don't use props is to get all the students to use the props so that they can see, for instance, how blocks can make the posture more challenging but help to avoid contorting the body to fit the pose.

'Props are only required to make the postures easier'

Using props can make certain postures easier to achieve, such as Trikonasana. There is nothing wrong with this – that is one of their many purposes. However, it should be noted that blocks can be used to make some asanas more challenging. For example, I often do Bakasana on blocks to demonstrate how they challenge my balance. Props have become my best friends, and one of the things I do when starting a new course is to recommend that my students invest in props.

As noted in other chapters, in a body positive class you should take each pose in stages. When demonstrating the various stages of a pose, you can offer a prop as an aid for all variations of the poses, reminding students that props are not just for beginners. For instance, in Bakasana the feet can be placed against the wall to provide support, or those who wish to make the pose more challenging can place blocks beneath the hands.

9

Consent and Touch

The topic of consent and touch is being more widely discussed by the yoga community than ever before, which is a positive step. When I started practising yoga I don't recall ever being asked for my consent when receiving an adjustment or touch, and this appeared to be the norm. It wasn't something that was really taught or talked about on my trainings either. A lot of teachers would have been taught about applying adjustments, but not about the potential implications of causing harm or trauma. I suppose it was always assumed that it would be okay to do so.

However, things have changed. As well as wider awareness around consent following the #metoo movement, a number of scandals within the yoga world have come to light. In recent years we have been hearing about abuse in various industries and, unfortunately, the yoga world is not exempt. *Practice and All Is Coming: Abuse, Cult Dynamics, and Healing in Yoga and Beyond* by Matthew Remski (2019a) mainly covers the abuse by Ashtanga founder Pattabhi Jois and how it was enabled. There have also been a number of other high-profile scandals in recent years.

The #yogatoo movement also brings to light the dynamic of spiritual abuse (Remski, 2019b). We must all take a moment to question how abuse has been enabled in so many schools of yoga, sometimes for many years. Has this been enabled because of the guru–student relationship, where power dynamics come into play, which could potentially allow abuse to take place? As yoga teachers we need, where possible, to ensure that this does not happen again and ask ourselves how we can work as a community to overcome these abuses of power and trust. Where was the ahimsa (non-harming) in the practice? Was it an abuse of power under the guise of adjustments? I am not here to corroborate these stories, but I believe it is an essential subject to discuss, especially if we are trying to create safe, judgement-free spaces and to guard against a repeat of this happening again. How were these gurus able to carry out these abuses unchecked?

When it comes to consent and touch during a class, it needs to be reinforced that the students are their own best teachers, and we are only there to guide and hold space for them – or should we perhaps consider this a collaboration? Imagine a new student who turns up to class unaware that they may be touched by someone they don't know (you!). Although this may not be an issue for some and might be seen as a welcome bonus, others may view it as receiving unwanted attention, which may be triggering or traumatic. A touch can, in some cases, trigger a memory of harm, causing the yoga practice to no longer feel safe and instead become a scary activity that potentially dysregulates the student. This is certainly not the reaction we wish to have.

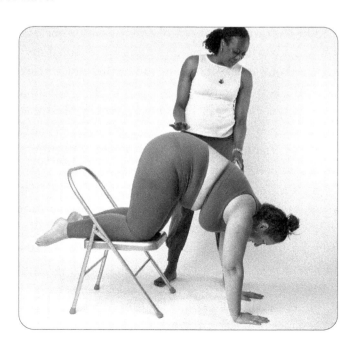

Touch/adjustments

In what is to be our 'new normal' due to COVID-19, hands-on adjustments may no longer be possible for the foreseeable future. As teachers, we are going to have to change the way we teach.

Adjustments should not be given by default. Teachers should be asking:

- Is the adjustment necessary?
- What is the purpose of the adjustment?
- What benefit will the student receive, if any?
- Are we making the adjustment because that's how we were taught during training?
- Are we able to cue the adjustment verbally instead?

We need to ascertain what experience is provided when we offer adjustments. Has it made the student's experience better or worse? Has permission to give the adjustment been received? So many questions, I hear you say!

I believe that the purpose of an adjustment is to aid a student's understanding of their practice. Adjustments are not supposed to be a way for us to impose our will on the student or to manipulate their body in order to make a posture look a certain way. When teaching yoga, it is very important to be able to recognise whether offering an adjustment is absolutely essential. In all classes there will be a variety of bodies, so it's going to be difficult to offer a 'one fits all' adjustment – I don't believe that such a thing exists. The purpose of yoga is not for us to fit our body to a pose, it's about yoga accommodating our bodies. I tend to offer a variety of ways for students to achieve each posture and leave it to them to decide what feels good.

Each posture will look different for everyone, and this should be expected. So offering an adjustment to accommodate a particular 'correct shape' (if such a shape existed) could potentially lead to injury. Remember – all bodies are unique!

Before you offer an adjustment, I suggest asking yourself the following:

- How will the adjustment make a difference to the experience of the pose?
- Will it actually help the student to achieve the pose in an easier or more accessible way?
- Most importantly, are you adequately trained to offer the adjustment?

If the answer is 'no' to any of these questions, then I suggest letting the student have agency over their body. Their body will be their best teacher.

Don't take it personally if a student doesn't want an assist or adjustment – we do not know their history. Be sure to let them know that it's also okay to tell you if they've changed their mind. It's not about us, or how we feel the posture should look – it's about the students, and we should make them feel they are in control.

Don't be afraid to stop an adjustment if you don't feel that it's appropriate or achieving what was intended. I have heard of instances where an adjustment has been offered which has unfortunately resulted in the student becoming injured. Keeping your students safe should be the number-one priority in class, and we should be mindful of this when offering adjustments at all times and take due care, no matter how well intentioned our actions. Students trust us and we should never cause them harm, whether physical or mental.

If it's found that an adjustment is indeed necessary and the student is happy to receive it, we need to obtain feedback from the student as to whether they felt better or worse following it. I've experienced loads of adjustments from teachers, but have rarely been asked if the adjustment made a difference to the pose (i.e. if the pose felt better or worse after the adjustment).

New students will not necessarily understand that they may be touched or receive hands-on adjustments during class. This is a side of yoga that is very rarely depicted on social media. Some may welcome this added bonus, but for others, it may be distracting or uncomfortable and even triggering. First, teachers don't know much about the students, they can't assume that it's okay to make adjustments. Second, to suddenly feel a touch when it's unexpected could potentially startle the student, affecting them mentally and physically even if they had previously indicated that they were okay with adjustments. Try to remain in their sight whenever possible.

Consider offering verbal adjustments – this is something I learnt when teaching general classes. You may find that a number of the other students will automatically make the suggested adjustment if they feel it is appropriate to their practice.

Consent

Consent is a dialogue that both parties have to agree to...or it can't be deemed as consent. As we are aware, emotions or feelings can change and therefore it's our responsibility to obtain consent for adjustments not only at the start of each class, but throughout the session.

I obtain consent discreetly during Savasana at the start of the class by asking students to raise their hands if they do not want to have an adjustment or to be touched. In addition to this, teachers need to be aware that some students may find it difficult to say no. Where possible, try to observe their body language to ascertain that it is congruent with the permission they gave. Remember, people come to yoga for different reasons, but one of the main ones is to feel safe and to enjoy the healing benefits of the practice, reinforcing why choice is so important.

Below are some ways in which to obtain consent.

Consent cards take the guesswork out of the tricky scenario of whether to touch or not touch. They're a very simple and clever concept that can help create a powerful experience for students, who can discreetly flip the consent card to indicate yes or no. Consent cards may not be ideal in all scenarios, for instance when teaching visually impaired students, or those doing a chair-based yoga practice as the card may be hard to reach.

We need to manage student expectations and ensure that students are aware that a 'yes' card does not necessarily mean they will receive an adjustment – for instance, we may run out of time or we may not wish to adjust everyone. Due to the COVID-19 pandemic, touch may no longer be permissible. If it is eventually reintroduced, be aware that people may still not feel comfortable being touched after a prolonged period of social distancing.

Consent cards don't have to be expensive. You can use regular playing cards or you can be creative and design your own.

Asking students individually if they'd like to be adjusted is another option as you navigate the yoga room. This gives you the opportunity to offer spontaneous adjustments. If you use this method, look at the student's body language and ask yourself whether they really seem to mean yes or are just trying to be polite.

Using your intuition can also be an option in cases where you have built up a relationship with a student who regularly allows you to adjust their practice. Nevertheless, still check and obtain permission, as it should never be assumed.

A yoga class is an energy exchange between the student and the teacher, and this should be respected. We really don't know a student's history and what emotional baggage they may be bringing into the yoga room. We should honour and respect the students' bodies in the same way that we ask them to honour their own bodies.

10

Yoga Sequences

Having an understanding of postures is a good basis from which to provide creative adaptations. You can do this by dissecting each pose and finding ways to make it accessible. It's always good to have a plan of the sequences you wish to teach, but be prepared to go off script, as you never know who is going to be in the room. Remember, it's not about the students adapting their bodies for the postures – it's about adapting the postures for their bodies.

Here are some traditional yoga poses with variations that help make them accessible so that you will be able to accommodate the variety of bodies that practise yoga. Use these poses as a starting point to evolve the practice so that more people will be inspired to get on the mat. Try out these options for yourself, and be creative!

Chair Surya Namaskar (chair sun salutation)

The classic Surya Namaskar can be done as a seated practice. This alternative can make this ubiquitous sequence more accessible for those who do not wish to do a floor-based practice.

If the feet cannot reach the floor, then blocks or blankets can be placed beneath the feet.

- From a seated position inhale and bring the hands together in prayer position in front of the chest.

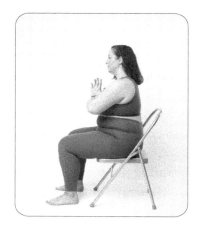

- Extend the hands up towards the ceiling and gently gaze straight ahead or up towards the hands.

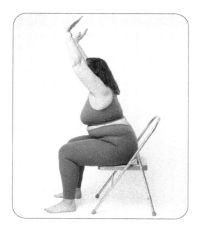

- Bring the hands down onto the thighs.

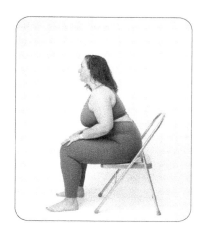

- While exhaling slowly, take the arms down and place them close to the feet.

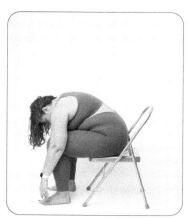

- Inhale and lift up the torso, to sit straight on the chair. Exhale, and lift the right leg up, and hold the right thigh with the hands while bending the knee.
- Inhale and press the thigh towards the chest, while bending the right knee in seated low lunge chair variation.

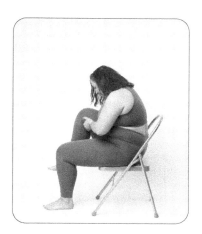

– Exhale and place the foot on the floor while stretching the arms above the head.

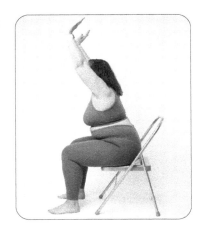

– Inhale and lift the arms up.
– Exhale and fold the torso forward over the thighs to come into forward fold.

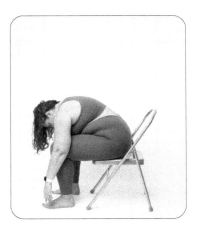

– Inhale and bend the left leg at the knee, bringing the thighs close to the body while seated straight in seated low lunge.

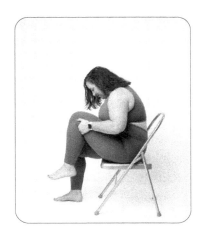

- Exhale and release the leg to the floor and fold forward. Slide the hands down towards the feet. Allow the head to relax.

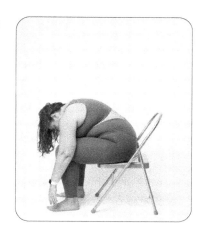

- Inhale and raise the hands over the head, keeping the spine straight.

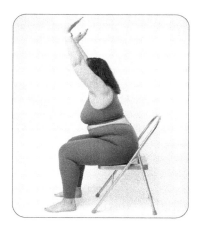

- Exhale and lower the hands to prayer position in front of the chest.

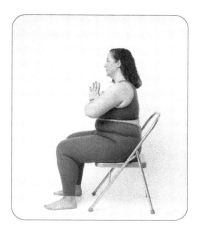

Balasana (child's pose)

Balasana is often described as a resting pose but it may not be a relaxing pose for everyone. There are a number of ways to allow this posture to be more comfortable and accessible in order to accommodate various body types.

- Start by kneeling on the floor and place a folded blanket under the knees for support. Knees can be wide apart or close together, whatever allows the student to feel most comfortable.
- The arms can be extended forward if the student wishes to do so.

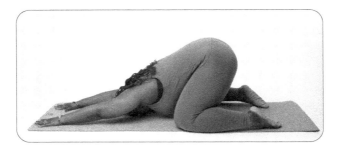

Chair variation

- While kneeling, face the seat of the chair and separate the knees to allow plenty of space for the body.
- Place the arms on the chair and fold them, grabbing opposite elbows if it feels comfortable. Lean forward with a straight spine and rest the head on the forearms.

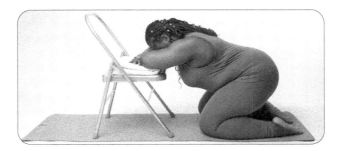

Balasana with a block or bolster

- Start in a kneeling position. Place a block or bolster on the floor or mat. The feet can be parallel, or wider to accommodate the body, with the top of the feet flat on the floor.
- Separate the knees as wide as possible to create space for the body when leaning forward.
- Start to lean forward and rest on the block or bolster. Find a comfortable position or turn the head to one side to rest it comfortably.
- The arms can be extended forward if the student wishes to do so.

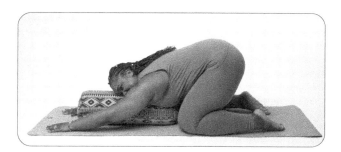

Balasana on the back

Alternatively, you can change the orientation of the pose and do Balasana on the back. Keeping the legs together or apart, or wider to accommodate the body, bend the knees and gently hug them towards the chest.

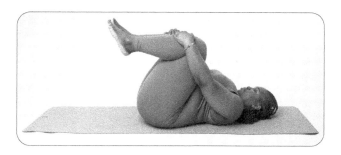

Eka Pada Rajakapotasana (pigeon pose)

Eka Pada Rajakapotasana has many accessible variations.

Floor-based Eka Pada Rajakapotasana, using a chair

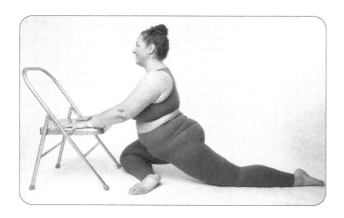

- Facing towards the seat of the chair, start on all fours. Place the hands on the seat of the chair.
- Bend the right knee and place it in front of the leg of the chair to your right. The right ankle is behind the leg of the chair to your left.
- The left leg should be extended behind so that the left knee is flat on the floor.
- The right hip should go back and left hip forward, to help keep the hips aligned.
- Walk the hands forward so that they can be extended. Keep the spine upright.
- Repeat on the other side.

Seated Eka Pada Rajakapotasana, on a chair

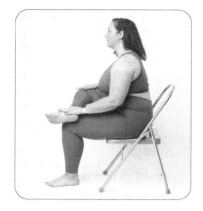

- Sit on a chair, a little forward so as not to lean into the back of the chair. The ankles should be directly below the knees. If the feet don't reach the floor, blocks can be used to raise the floor to allow a connection.
- Bring your right knee towards the chest and give it a good hug.
- With the knee bent, flex the right foot and begin to drop the knee open to the right by rotating the thigh outward from the hip joint.
- Rest the right ankle on the left thigh, just above the left knee.
- Alternatively, stretch the left leg straight with the heel on the floor, and rest the right ankle lower down the left leg, which can help to avoid pain.
- If you can feel a deep stretch sitting up tall, then stay here. If not, hold onto the seat of the chair and breathe in to lengthen the spine. Fold forward from the hip creases, keeping the spine long to begin with. Only go as far as is comfortable, then allow the spine to gently round to get an extra back stretch.
- Stay where you are and breathe. Send the breath down to the belly and the right outer hip, and breathe out to release and soften as much as you can.
- Repeat on the other side.

Standing Eka Pada Rajakapotasana, using a chair

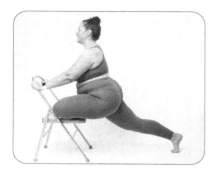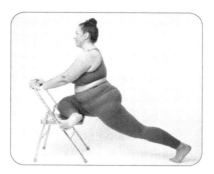

- Stand in front of the seat of the chair.
- While holding onto the back of the chair, bend one knee, lifting the foot off the floor, and as you externally rotate the thigh, place the shin and thigh on the seat of the chair.
- Slide the free leg behind you until it is fully extended.
- The toes can be tucked to get more of a calf stretch, or place the top of the foot on the floor for a deeper ankle and shin stretch.
- Keep the arms straight and lengthen the spine.
- Repeat on the other side.

Chair Bakasana (chair crow pose)

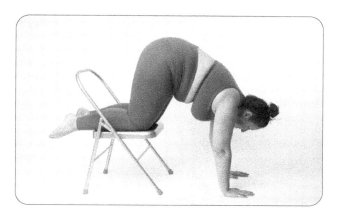

- Start by kneeling on the chair seat facing forward. The feet should be together and knees apart.
- Carefully place the hands the floor, so that the hands can be directly underneath the shoulders. If this is not possible, blocks can be placed on the floor in front of the legs of the chair, helping to raise the floor. The hips should be directly above the knees or adjusted as needed.
- When the pose is completed keep the hands on the floor or blocks and then place one foot on the floor at a time.

Adho Mukha Svanasana (downward-facing dog)

Adho Mukha Svanasana is a posture that is often described as a resting posture in the same way that Balasana is, but unfortunately this is not the case for everyone.

Suggested cueing:

- Ensure that students are sufficiently warmed up before attempting Adho Mukha Svanasana.
- Start on all fours, on your hands and knees in table-top position.
- The wrists can be slightly in front of the shoulders. The hands should be shoulder-width apart or a little wider. Press the fingers and palms of the hands firmly into the floor.
- Spread the fingers as wide as possible, with the index finger facing forward.
- The knees should be hip-width apart with the knees directly under the hips, the lower legs pointing straight back from the knees; tops of feet should be flat on the floor.
- You may need to rotate the top of the arms so that the inside creases (eyes) of the elbows face the opposite corner of each mat. This will broaden the collarbone. Try to ensure that the hands are still pressing into the floor.
- Tuck the toes under and start to lift the knees off the floor. Lift the hips up to the ceiling.
- There's the option to pedal the feet a few times by bending then straightening the knees, first the right and then the left.
- Keep the arms and the spine as straight as possible. There is the option to have a micro bend in the knees.
- Try to ensure that students have an awareness of the upper body. The hands should continue to actively push the floor away. The shoulders are drawn away from the ears to ensure that tension is released.
- Stay here for two breaths, before allowing the knees to come back down to the floor and coming into Balasana.

When students are new to yoga, they may not be able to distribute the weight correctly. This can place pressure on the wrists and hands, resulting in potential pain or sensations in them. This will invariably disappear over time with practice. Remember, it is not about being perfect, it is about the practice helping to build and cultivate strength in the body.

Further discomfort for students with curvy bodies may come about for those who may be abundant in the breast area, as this may cause additional weight to be placed on the wrists and hands. If this is the case, ensure the student's hands are pressed firmly into the floor with each index finger facing forward. Pressing the thumb and index finger into the floor will remove pressure from the wrist.

Using props

Another option to alleviate this problem is the use of blocks under the hands, which helps to shift the centre of gravity so that the weight shifts towards the legs.

- Place two blocks at the front of the mat approximately shoulder-width apart.
- Place the hands on the blocks, and lift the knees off the floor as the hips move towards the ceiling. The knees can remain bent or straighten to suit the student's preference.
- Ensure the student's hands are pressed firmly into the blocks with their index fingers facing forward. This removes the pressure from the wrist.

If the student still feels pain, suggest placing a towel beneath the base of the hands in order to help shift the weight forward – helping to change the angle of the hands. You can also use wedges that have been specifically designed for this purpose.

Another option is to do Adho Mukha Svanasana at the wall to avoid bearing weight on the hands. Begin by standing close to the wall and pressing the hands against the wall at around hip height.

Gradually step the feet away from the wall, keeping the hands in place, until the arms are straight.

Forearm variation

If none of the above suggestions make the posture feel more comfortable, forearm dog is worth exploring. This variation is a good way for students to start to gain confidence and build strength in the arms before graduating to Adho Mukha Svanasana.

- Start on all fours and prepare in the same way as for Adho Mukha Svanasana.
- Blocks can be placed between the hands to help with the correct placement of the forearms. Press the forearms into the floor.
- Tuck the toes under and lift the hips up in the same way as for Adho Mukha Svanasana.

Chaturanga Dandasana (four-limbed staff pose)

Chaturanga is another ubiquitous pose, which forms part of the Surya Namaskar sequence. Students can find it challenging as it requires a lot of upper body strength when the body is being lowered towards the floor. I have found when teaching Chaturanga that most students will be willing to work with a variation that can be adapted depending on how they feel. Over time the students will gain confidence in this posture and won't feel self-conscious. I continually state that they should not worry about how the posture looks and remind them to be patient and keep practising. The fear associated with Chaturanga is not having enough strength or control to support the body and invariably being worried about how they look while trying to do the pose.

Here are some variations that will help students to build the required strength in the core and upper body in ways that will provide the required support and confidence. When students feel ready or more confident, they may wish to try Chaturanga without any props.

Chaturanga using blocks

- Come onto all fours and place a block beneath the chest. Get the students to experiment with using the side and end of the block to ascertain what works best for them.
- The elbows should be bent to approximately 90 degrees, so the students are able to rest the sternum on the block while having the option of keeping the knees bent or straight.

Chaturanga using a bolster

- Place a bolster on the floor, then come into plank or a modified plank (knees on the floor). The knees are behind the hips, and the wrists are below the shoulders.
- Slowly lower the body onto the bolster. Push the floor away

and keep the elbows pointing towards the back of room as the body is lowered onto the bolster.

- The beauty here is that the bolster supports the weight of the body.

Chaturanga using the wall

This version is good for starting to help build the strength required in Chaturanga.

- Start facing the wall. Students should place the arms in front of them at chest height, with the palms touching the wall. Come into a modified plank position, with the feet behind the hips.
- Press the hands against the wall and step the feet forward a little, then lower the body towards the wall – bending the arms at the elbow (in a similar way that would be done on the mat version).

Transitions

One of the most challenging transitions for students is the step through. This normally takes place when students are stepping forward from Adho Mukha Svanasana into a lunge. The reason for this challenge is that parts of the body, like the abdomen, may get in the way. Placing blocks under the hands will create space, but another option is to allow the student to step the foot wide and come into the forward fold via a wide lunge. For example, if the right foot is stepping forward it can be placed outside of the right hand. Another option is to lift up the right hand as the foot is being stepped forward, again creating space. There are no limits to the number of steps taken to bring the foot forward, so ensure the students know they can take as many steps as is necessary, demonstrating that everyone's practice is unique and their own.

The beauty of yoga and its poses is that as it's always evolving and becoming more accessible, there is a style of yoga for everybody. We just need to help potential students find the right one for them.

BE CREATIVE

Take the time to explore some common yoga postures to see how you can adapt them for different bodies and levels of experience. For example, you could think about creative variations of the following poses:

- Garudasana
- Trikonasana
- Paschimottanasana.

Keep in mind the following points:

- What props can you use to make the posture more accessible for people with different body shapes, and people with various injuries or conditions?
- Can you use a different orientation of the pose to make it more accessible (hint: if a standing pose is tricky because of an injury or due to issues with balance, the student could try it, lying down on their front or back, or seated)?
- Think about the various stages and elements of each pose and break them down to find a version that the student can do. When you think you have the simplest version of a pose, question whether you can make it even more accessible. Challenge yourself!

Remember, try not to avoid postures just because they might feel 'difficult' – instead try and find a variation of the pose that works for the person practising it so that they can benefit from it.

Part 3

BODY POSITIVITY OFF THE YOGA MAT

II

Body Positive Yoga
off the Mat

*A yoga that doesn't hold social justice at its
heart is not a complete or true yoga.*

Lakshmi Nair, Satya Yoga Cooperative

In this chapter we will look at Health at Every Size® (HAES®), an approach that challenges the notion of weight loss as a health goal, and how it can help address biased views both on and off the mat, especially around diet culture. We'll also explore how social justice is at the core of yoga and the body positive movement, and how these relate to ahimsa (non-violence for ourselves and others). When these intersect, there are, I believe, political connotations, which can change the ways in which we potentially interact with society. This was certainly my experience, so much so that I left behind all the things society told me that I wanted after committing to the yoga path. Spiritual bypassing is also explored to show how it is sometimes used as a way of avoiding discussing difficult experiences and situations like discrimination in terms of age, size, ethnicity or disability.

Body positive yoga has made me question some long-held views and go back to the original teachings of yoga. Real yoga takes place off the mat and is integrated into our lives: it is how we interact and support others – it is yoga in action, it is being the change we wish to see in the world. As I said earlier, we are all born yogis. It's only as we grow that we start to lose this connection to yoga in our lives.

Body positive yoga comprises so many elements that allow us to reconnect to yoga, take it off the mat and incorporate it into daily life. Yoga does not have to involve an asana – simply lying on your mat and breathing (i.e. pranayama/breath control) is yoga. But it's also a way of living, a way of being and a way of being aware.

Health at Every Size® (HAES®)

I believe that yoga can be transformational for everyone. Living in a society rife with stereotypes and stigma concerning bodies that do not conform to what is considered the ideal can be deeply damaging, but yoga can help to challenge these long-held views. It offers a relief from trauma and the chance to reconnect with ourselves, as it's about seeing the body from the inside out, rather than solely from the outside. Yoga's role is to teach us to realise our bodies' true potential and to cultivate self-acceptance and eventually self-love for our bodies as they are. I appreciate that this can be difficult, as we might not love our body every single day – it's okay for a self-acceptance journey to take time. Making peace with the body results in greater confidence and living a more engaged life, as we begin to honour our bodies for all the things they can do and not punish them for what they can't.

Being aware of the Health at Every Size® ethos is one way we can educate ourselves and end the pressure to make bodies small through diets. Learning about HAES® and its place in yoga has underpinned the phrase that I like to use so much: 'every body is a yoga body'. Continuing our education helps us to help students to cultivate self-acceptance and possibly self-love as we address concerns around the idealised 'yoga body' and remove any biases that may be held about body shapes and sizes. As discussed elsewhere in this book, health is a complex subject based on many factors, but unfortunately, body size and weight are seen as indicators of health within much of the wellness space, resulting in discrimination. Although of course weight loss can be a by-product of adopting a healthy lifestyle, it's not necessarily an indicator of one.

AN EXAMPLE OF DISCRIMINATION

Here's an example of a time I decided to share a picture of myself and another yogi, Jessica, to demonstrate that yoga is for everyone, regardless of size or shape. This picture garnered very positive reactions and inspired potential yogis to get on the mat. However, when I shared it in a UK teachers' Facebook group, I was astounded at the negative reaction. The comments did not focus on the beauty of the postures and what they represented; instead they focused on weight and someone's body without any knowledge of their medical history. This was disappointing, to say the least. The two yogis were simply sharing their practice in ways that were accessible for their bodies.

I felt so strongly about the dissent and visceral comments I received that I issued a statement that outlined my stance on body positive yoga and posted it within the group.

The HAES® movement can be traced back to the 1960s, when it advocated the view that the changing culture towards beauty standards was having negative health and psychological repercussions for fat people (https://en.wikipedia.org/wiki/Health_at_Every_Size).

The HAES® framework supports health, wellbeing, eating and movement and is committed to dismantling systemic oppression (in the form of sizeism and fat phobia). It was established in 2003 by the Association of Size Diversity and Health. It rejects the idea that BMI, size or weight should be considered a significant factor in determining health. Weight can be one of many indications of health, but it should not be the sole one. The key factors behind HAES® are:

- **Weight inclusivity:** The diversity of body sizes and shapes is respected and accepted. Any idealisation of specific weights is rejected.
- **Health enhancement:** Support the promotion of health

initiatives that will help improve equity and access to services and practices that will enhance wellbeing, for example, economic, social, physical and emotional.

- **Respectful care:** Acknowledgement of our biases will help work towards ending biases and discrimination pertaining to weight. The provision of services and information that will create understanding of how racialised identity, gender, age, socio-economic and other factors can have an impact on weight stigma and support ways in which these inequities are addressed.
- **Eating for wellbeing:** Promote individualised eating that is flexible, and based on hunger, nutritional requirements and pleasure, rather than on diets that focus on weight control.
- **Life-enhancing movement:** Support physical activities that allow people of diverse sizes, abilities and interests to participate in movements they find enjoyable and that can be adapted.

(adapted from Association for Size Diversity and Health, 2020)

I discovered the HAES® framework early on in my body positive journey, although recently it's being embraced more and more in the mainstream. It resonated with what I was starting to believe as it provides a different perspective on health and wellbeing. It was so refreshing to find something challenging the diet culture rhetoric. HAES® seeks to move away from the emphasis on weight loss as a health goal, educate on the stigma faced by people who are considered overweight, and reduce the stigma.

Body positive yoga can use the HAES® framework and messages to tackle these issues, both on the mat, in terms of making us appreciate our bodies and all they can do, and off the mat. One way I do this is by sharing diverse images on my social media platforms so that all bodies become normalised. #YogaHasNoSize is one of my favourite terms, and I use it to promote inclusion to show any future students that size does not matter and should not stop anyone from starting a yoga practice. I must be becoming boring now by saying that yoga does not discriminate; it is the teachers who do. But for the purpose of this book, it's important that YOU break this pattern. Be aware of unconscious biases and the discrimination and barriers facing your potential students so that these can be addressed.

Diet culture and HAES®

The HAES® message seeks to dispel diet culture, which is steeped in racism, patriarchy and white supremacy. Unfortunately diet culture is creeping into the yoga space, as diet and health have become intertwined – we now have to untangle this scenario. It can be difficult for the wellbeing or fitness industry to understand the philosophy of HAES®, as individuals may not understand the underlying causes of weight issues or may hold outdated views (e.g. they often believe that simply going on a diet will solve the issue of weight, when other factors may be involved). Determining someone's health status based solely on their weight can have a detrimental effect. For instance, I have colleagues who were not employed by some gyms because their size was considered a deterrent for clients – as their body should be 'aspirational'. There is a lot of pressure on teachers to look a certain way, and this is becoming problematic as it is making them question whether yoga is for them. I have also heard of teachers – who may have eating disorders – bringing their views about food and diets into their classes. This cannot be a good combination, especially if it goes unchecked and unacknowledged.

WHAT IS DIET CULTURE?

Diet culture encompasses messages that make us believe we are not good enough in the bodies that we have, and that we would be happier, more worthwhile and valuable if our bodies were different.

Diet culture becomes a cycle, because diets do not work. If they did, then why is the diet industry worth an estimated $71 billion (£53.6 billion) annually in the US, and growing every year? (Lau, 2021).

We are being told that if we want to fit in and be happy, we need to lose weight and be thin, and if we 'fail' then it's our fault for being somehow 'weak'. But I've heard from many people who have become entangled in this cycle who have reached this goal (of thinness) only to say that they haven't achieved happiness and have instead found themselves with disordered eating. We are now hearing about 'clean eating', 'intermittent fasting' and 'good' and 'bad' foods, which some believe are different forms of diets, but as the saying goes, a leopard never changes its spots.

Are some of us addicted to food or addicted to dieting? To answer this, as with most things, we need to look at the root cause and not just stick a temporary plaster over the proverbial wound. When we are continually and unconsciously surrounded with messaging that tells us we need to change, it's little wonder that we feel the need to do so. However, what we actually need is inside every single one of us.

Diet culture can and often does lead to eating disorders and, just as in yoga, marginalised groups can be made invisible – it is not only people with thin, white bodies who have this problem. It is a mental health issue.

I am very much against diet culture because of what it stands for. We must remember that the body is an amazing vessel or, as some like to say, a temple, and it essentially does what it needs to do. Our body knows best, which is why I believe in intuitive eating – a philosophy where you make peace with all food types. It requires us to stop looking at food as 'good' or 'bad'. Essentially you are the expert on your body and its hunger signals – listening to the body and eating what feels good for the body.

If anyone uses the body positivity message to promote diet culture in any way, this is unethical, and you have to question their motivations as this is not what body positivity is about. There is also absolutely no diet talk in my classes, because I do not know what someone is going through or what their relationship with food is. I do share aspects of my life, but I am very careful about the things I talk about in class. Our role is to make our students feel they will be accepted just as they are, and diet culture is just one of many barriers to participation. For us, as teachers, creating a safe, judgement-free space for students to have advocacy over their bodies is an important role.

One film about the diet industry that I really recommend is *Embrace* by body-image activist Taryn Brumfitt (Brumfitt, 2016). She explores the global issue of body loathing and aims to inspire us to change the way we feel about our bodies and ourselves, so that we gain an insight into how we absorb all the unconscious messages of how our bodies need to be fixed.

HAES® focuses on promoting social, playful and pleasurable movement, which includes dancing, cycling and exercise, and activities associated with everyday life, such as walking and gardening. Movement is encouraged for the purpose of enjoyment, involvement in a community and improved quality of life. This is an excellent example of taking yoga off the mat. Remember, yoga should not be a punishment – it should be a practice of love for your body.

Other ways of taking yoga off the mat

The practice of yoga does not end when we roll up our mats at the end of class; in fact, this is when the real yoga begins, as we take what we've learnt into our everyday lives. The way I teach yoga provides tools that help my students every day. First, I break it down so that students can change any misconceptions that they have that yoga is solely about the asana. I often start by asking how getting your leg behind your head can help you in your everyday life. This normally gets a lot of laughter before the question hits home. Then I explain that merely being on the mat and breathing can inform you of how you are feeling, and allow you to tune into the body's messages. We often underestimate the power of the breath, and its importance; we can do without water for a few days and food for a few weeks, but what will happen if we don't breathe? I remember reading on social media that one of my teacher training buddies had been in a bank when a robbery took place, and her breath got her through the situation – she could connect to it to stop her body from reacting to this scary situation. She was also able to help the other customers to keep calm and avoid any further danger. This is the magic of yoga.

Yoga off the mat can be so many things for different people. Yoga allowed me to heal from Bell's palsy, and it can profoundly affect people's lives in numerous ways. Yoga is my medicine, or sometimes I say it is my WD-40 as it allows me to become flexible not only in my body but also in my mind. The physical practice of yoga is medicine for our bodies and our hearts. It can allow you to become more conscious as you come off autopilot, and become aware of all the beauty in life around you. It can also give you clarity so that you realise what's important to you and that you are the director of your life, not just an actor. It allows you to care more about your environment and how we leave it for future generations. The skills we learn on the mat can turn into transferable practices such as tolerance, the ability to let go of things that are no longer serving us well, love, patience, kindness and compassion.

I love the saying 'You can practise a week of yoga without doing a single asana, and this too is yoga' (source unknown). It demonstrates so eloquently that yoga is more than just asanas. But another way to perceive this is that we are doing yoga every single day off the mat. Yoga is life.

We rely on the body's inherent wisdom for all things. We are made this way, but there is a point when this changes, when we actively try to stop listening to the body's innate wisdom and instead start to adhere to societal expectations and conditioning. All bodies are beautiful, and we need to learn to appreciate them more, not for how they look but for all the amazing things they do for us without us even asking.

THE YAMAS AND NIYAMAS

For many, like myself, yoga has become a way of life and expanded outside of what I practise in the yoga room. What can start as a form of exercise can grow into something much more as we try to integrate yoga's teachings into our everyday lives by following the Yamas and Niyamas (a series of ethical rules). This allows the real yoga to happen, when you can take yoga off the mat and out into your everyday life. The Yamas and Niyamas, which are the first two steps of the eight limbs of yoga, are often described as ethical or moral codes that can help us navigate life more consciously, and which yogis are taught to embrace or abide by. In my experience many students are not initially aware of Yamas and Niyamas or the eight limbs. The limbs consist of Yamas, Niyamas, Asana, Pranayama, Pratyahara, Dharana, Dhyana and Samadhi. Note that Asana (physical yoga poses) is not the first limb, but the third.

Below is a list of their definitions:

1. **Yamas:** How we interact with others. They are expressed as five moral constraints:
   - ahimsa (non-harming)
   - satya (truthfulness)
   - asteya (non-stealing)
   - bramacharya (moderation)
   - aparigraha (generosity).
2. **Niyamas:** How we relate to ourselves:
   - santosa (contentment)
   - tapas (self-discipline)
   - svadhyaya (self-study)
   - isvara pranidhana (surrender to the divine)
   - saucha (cleanliness).
3. **Asanas:** The postures practised in yoga. The purpose of the yoga posture is to help develop focus and concentration, allowing the practitioner to master the body in preparation for meditations (which may result in long periods of sitting).
4. **Pranayama:** Breath control. Breathing techniques designed to help channel or control the prana (life-force energy),

allowing awareness of the breath to help calm and create self-awareness.

5. **Pratyahara:** Withdrawal of the senses, where practitioners withdraw from the external world to connect with their inner landscape. Moving away from external distractions so that we can connect with our innate wisdom.

6. **Dharana:** Concentration. After removing ourselves from external distractions, the mind can be focused on an idea or on an object.

7. **Dhyana:** Uninterrupted awareness. Whereas Dharana is one-pointed attention, Dhyana is being fully aware or mindful without focus. The experience is one of wide-open consciousness, effortless and calm.

8. **Samadhi:** Often referred to as enlightenment, this is the ultimate goal of yoga. Connection with everything where we all become one, there being no separation between all living beings.

It's also important to note that with the exception of the last three limbs, the eight limbs of yoga do not need to be practised in any particular order. They are all interconnected and non-exclusive, and each helps cultivate the development of the others.

The benefits of being mindful

Apart from the physical aspects of yoga, practising being mindful is just one way that yoga is so beneficial. The power of being mindful of the body and the self should not be underestimated. Being mindful means that we are conscious. We then have the capacity to listen to our bodies, and respond intuitively to their needs. Practising being present and conscious on the mat enables us to transfer this consciousness into our daily lives. We are then able to tap into the innate wisdom of the body, and it becomes normal to do things intuitively – moving, eating and resting intuitively. Rather than listening to the external noises from family, friends and society, we become more trusting of our own wisdom and decisions. We can then perform self-study and discover our own truths and unconscious biases.

As part of one of my first yoga trainings, for a period of two weeks, I was asked to remove meat from my diet, refrain from watching TV, and to journal daily. This request indicated to me that I was experiencing yoga in a way that was so much more than just the asana. Yoga became part of every aspect of my daily life. The impact it made on me was huge; as well as becoming more present, I also saw that I was capable of so much more than I realised. By gaining more time to actively and mindfully engage with the world and becoming more connected with myself than ever before, I realised that I was able to be creative; I even made a leather journal with the OM symbol on the front, which I was so proud of. When I later visited India and spent time at Akhanda Ashram, I was able to be of service and do the tasks I was allocated, much the same way as many yogis did thousands of years ago. It was a very humbling experience, showing me that I don't need all the trappings of life and can lead a very modest but happy existence.

I was able to take yoga off the mat by following my intuition and creating Curvesomeyoga. Little did I know that this was to be my path. Through the practice of ahimsa my goal was to share the benefits of yoga, innocently wanting to make yoga more inclusive and accessible as my way of being of service. Now I want to disrupt more of the status quo so that yoga and wellbeing for everybody is embraced in more of the world, resulting in collective liberation. Yoga has always had a body positive element. It's ultimately about personal liberation and then collective liberation; first, it frees us from the constraints of our upbringing and societal expectations, and then it makes us want to go out and promote greater equity and inclusion.

I like to think that I am now part of the collective liberation. This path has come about after adhering to my yoga practice, which incorporates the eight limbs of yoga. Although this wasn't apparent when I first started Curvesomeyoga, it's very much the case now. My purpose is to help create equity for those who are often invisible within the yoga community and beyond, to be of service and come from a place of love in a world where this is not always readily available, to unlearn so I can gain more incredible learnings and insights. This is social justice in action.

Reading the *Bhagavad Gita* (often referred to as the first book of yoga) during my yoga teacher training, I began to see how yoga is a reflection of life. The conversation between Krishna and Arjuna on the battlefield is a metaphor for our daily struggles as we make choices that start to challenge the societal norms or expectations. The *Gita* is unique in its message as it illustrates how we have to follow our purpose, our duty, to live and work in the world. Herein lies its ingenuity and continued relevance – the book demonstrates that social justice has always been an integral part of yoga. I didn't fully recognise this for many years, until I took part in training courses like Accessible Yoga, Yoga for Humankind and body positive yoga. How could a book that was written thousands of years ago still be so relevant?

Yoga is social justice

Yoga without social justice is spiritual bypassing.

Mei Lai Swan, Founder, Yoga for Humankind

The body positive movement in its previous iteration had a political stance, but this has been lost as it has become a trend that has been embraced by brands and used to make money. If your yoga has ahimsa at its core, it too is political and is steeped in social justice. If it doesn't, then I would ask that you seriously consider what yoga means to you.

What is ahimsa?

Ahimsa is commonly taken to mean 'non-violence', but more literally translated from Sanskrit as 'absence of injury' (www.yogajournal. com/lifestyle/what-is-ahimsa). If we're not practising ahimsa are we really practising yoga? I love Susanna Barkataki's question, posed on

Instagram: 'When I say practise, I don't mean are we being kind all the time...but are we *practising* being kind?' In this case we mean really trying, most likely failing (often), but always striving to be kind in our thoughts, words and actions. Do we practise ahimsa towards our families and friends; to acquaintances, strangers and those we disagree with or find difficult to understand; to the environment, animals and natural world; and to ourselves? Ahimsa can be as simple as being more aware of the language we use in our everyday life so that we carry the do-no-harm ethos with us.

Ahimsa is where social justice interacts with yoga. Practising ahimsa means we are actively working towards and committed to creating equity for everyone. This is what makes yoga potentially a political fight. An example of ahimsa is not ignoring a situation when a fellow teacher may be experiencing microaggressions and standing up for them. It took me some time to reflect and think about how I practise ahimsa – I try to practise ahimsa as a form of social justice by attempting to disrupt the yoga and wellbeing spaces so that there is greater equality and equity. By making yoga more inclusive, you can help to educate others on how their behaviour can help to reduce the harm that is being caused by our society in terms of the inequality and discrimination faced by marginalised groups.

The principle of ahimsa has had an enormous impact as a means to confront social and political injustice. Mohandas Gandhi successfully employed non-violent civil disobedience to free India from British imperialism; Martin Luther King Jr used non-violent resistance in the civil rights movement against discriminatory laws in the US. The principle of non-violence was also crucial in ending apartheid in South Africa. Globally, non-violent resistance is regularly employed as a peaceful means of protest to enact social and political change and an alternative to brutal confrontation. The organisation Off the Mat Into the World (www.offthematintotheworld.org) is a good resource for social justice. It's so heartening to see that so many others now want to create a more equitable world through yoga, and this can be validated by the increase in yoga and social justice teachings available. There are so many teachers and organisations that have social justice at the core of their teaching: Anusha Wijeyakumar, Jivana Heyman, Dr Lee

Watson (founder of the yoga community Fierce Calm) and Susanna Barkataki – I am pleased to say that there are too many to name.

If yoga doesn't hold social justice at its centre, how can it be real yoga? Many individuals, including myself, consider the omission of social justice from yoga to be a form of spiritual bypassing, as highlighted by Mei Lai Swan. So, consider this: if your yoga is solely about getting bodies on mats, much like burger chains are about getting bums on seats, and there's no philosophical change taking place, are you even practising yoga in the way it was intended? However, if your aim is to get students to try yoga, with the potential of deepening their physical practice – is there anything wrong with this? This requires deep contemplation.

I used to feel there was something not right with the gimmicky styles of yoga in terms of their authenticity. But I've seen so many yogis develop a relationship with yoga after those initial experiences, which has flourished and deepened their practice. It is not for me to determine if the styles deemed to be gimmicky are less valid – but if they open up the yoga space to people who would otherwise not practise yoga – is this wrong, even though some styles may seem far removed from the origins of yoga? It has to be remembered that many recent styles of yoga that were initially viewed in the same way, for example Acroyoga, Bikram and aerial yoga, have now become part of the mainstream. However, it should be noted it can be hard to find the yoga in some of the practices – maybe the word 'yoga' should be removed from their names.

People come to yoga for a multitude of reasons, many of them superficial, not least because the face of yoga that we see is the asana. But this doesn't mean that people will not soon come to understand the practice on a deeper level and start to live a more yogic life off their mats too.

Yoga is about the liberation of the many and not the few. It is about holding space for marginalised individuals and acknowledging the oppression experienced in our society. To do yoga is to help ensure that everyone has equal rights, and the access to healthcare, housing and education so often afforded to affluent individuals. But if this does not occur, how can this philosophy be said to be achieved?

We must really reflect on how our yoga aligns to the original teachings and keep them in mind both on and off the mat.

Spiritual bypassing

Spiritual bypassing is a 'tendency to use spiritual ideas and practices to sidestep or avoid facing unresolved emotional issues, psychological wounds, and unfinished developmental tasks' (Fossella and Welwood, 2011). The term was introduced in the early 1980s by John Welwood, a Buddhist teacher and psychotherapist. Welwood began to notice that people, including himself, would use spirituality as a defence mechanism to avoid working through hard emotions or confronting issues such as racism or discrimination, and would simply dismiss them with spiritual explanations. In light of the death of George Floyd and the BLM movement, I believe that there's been an awakening that has led to more open discussions on social media and elsewhere, where some of these difficult discussions around race have been able to take place.

In the case of yoga, this might look like wrapping the pain of racial trauma in tidier packaging so as to negate the significance of the discrimination experienced. Or it might manifest as a desire to only voice positive messages without acknowledging the truth or value of heightened emotions. Examples of spiritual bypassing that I've often heard are when people say, 'I don't see colour', 'love and peace', 'we are one', 'good vibes only' when responding to difficult situations. These often quick and glib responses do not acknowledge people's lived experience in a compassionate way and appear dismissive. Life is about balance, so that means positivity is not the solution for everything. Solely focusing on the positives is not feasible or realistic in all real-world scenarios. Lived experiences cannot be removed by saying 'love and light'.

Yoga philosophy says that we are all one, but it would be wrong to ignore the fact that there are differences in how people are treated and how they experience the world around them. In the world that we live in, to be considered one human race we would all have equal access to food, education, healthcare and jobs.

Spiritual bypassing perpetuates the idea that the belief 'we are one' is enough to create a reality where we are treated equally and as one. It is not. Spiritual bypassing permits the status quo to stay in place and teaches people that if you believe in something and have a good intent that is enough. It is not. (Johnson, 2020, p.31)

Spiritual bypassing can be very subtle and can often go unnoticed except by the person on the receiving end of such rebuttals. The idea behind some of these statements may seem nice or well intentioned in theory, but in fact they are problematic and can be viewed as ways in which to invalidate lived experiences.

So much harm and trauma can be caused by spiritual bypassing. As teachers, we need to put ourselves in the shoes of others. Just because we don't experience certain situations does not mean it's okay to ignore them or think that they don't exist. Acknowledgement is an impactful way to ensure that change occurs and that the space we hold is safe. Bringing compassion to the situation means that we are more open to listening and understanding. Also reflect on any preconceived ideas that you may have so that you are open to evaluating different perspectives. We see body positive yoga in action when we are able to better understand and appreciate the lived experiences of diverse groups.

Spiritual bypassing may seem like a new concept, so as teachers we need to take the time to understand it. Be open to discovering if you use any forms of spiritual bypassing in order to deal with uncomfortable or difficult situations. Always remember that it is okay to be imperfect as long as you are not coming from a place of harm. Sometimes, listening and learning to understand someone's lived experience will help, but be aware of instances where spiritual bypassing is taking place and be prepared to change in order to ensure that you are able to acknowledge their lived experience.

12

Conclusion

The future of body positive yoga

Yoga's future is bright but, more importantly, it is accessible.

The yoga landscape has changed beyond recognition recently, not least due to the COVID-19 pandemic. Literally overnight the majority of the yoga community had to move away from traditional in-person classes and start teaching online – resulting in the Zoom boom. Alongside this, there's a movement to ensure greater accessibility and inclusivity within yoga, including emerging conversations about body positivity, mental health, education and social justice. These forms of yoga have a foundation based on collective liberation, which is now seen a lot more frequently within the yoga community. It is essential that these conversations are taking place and helping to form the future of yoga. All of these changes have resulted in a very steep learning curve, which serves to demonstrate the overall resilience of the yoga and wellbeing communities.

Yoga will always have a place in our society, not just because of its broad reach but because of its transformational benefits. As its popularity continues to grow, we are now seeing yoga being prescribed by the medical profession as it's recognised as being part of a healthy lifestyle. As many in society are now turning to yoga to seek a more holistic way of life, so too are many seeing its benefits in terms of mental health, an issue that's being discussed more than I have ever seen – especially in light of the pandemic.

In this chapter, I offer some predictions on how yoga, particularly body positive yoga, will evolve. These stem from my experience, my yoga journey, and how yoga and its history intersect and relate to the modern world. The authors of the original yogic texts would not have been able to see how yoga would fit into modern times. Did they already know that yoga would stand the test of time? Although the practice was designed to grow and evolve, its roots also need to be respected and its important elements should not be removed.

Is the future online?

One benefit of the recent transition to online classes is that yoga has become more accessible to many potential practitioners – although it should be noted that some people have been excluded due to a lack of access to technology, or to a space to practise yoga, and so on. I believe that the move online will continue and know that this is something that I will personally continue. As we all start to embrace our 'new normal', a hybrid model is now available – a combination of in-person and online classes – giving students more choice than ever before. There are other benefits to students having the option to do online classes. Practising at home is a more convenient option for some, and removes a lot of students' perceived barriers to attending class. Online classes can provide students with more agency over their bodies as hands-on adjustments are not possible, and they may feel safer practising in their home environment. Having the choice to turn their camera on or not also means students are more empowered and have greater agency over their body in terms of not having to worry about adjustments or who can see their body. Another benefit to online classes is that students can access teachers who may not have been previously available to them. I found this in my own teaching: some students had wanted to practise with me but couldn't because of geographical constraints, but they are now able to attend my online classes.

Going back to yoga's roots

Recently, there seems to have been an awakening, where teachers like myself are starting to question their teachings and have begun a journey of unlearning, to relearn about yoga with a less Western perspective. Many are now seeking out other teachers for whom yoga has been part of their heritage and culture and who have a wealth of knowledge and experience. Having seen the disparities within the mainstream/commercial yoga space, they want to ensure that they are honouring the origins of yoga and, in turn, are able to offer classes that are both body positive and inclusive. Those who have become part of the body positive movement have seen how yoga has become distorted by capitalism, cultural appropriation and white supremacy, and are choosing instead to align with the original yogic teachings. The eight limbs of yoga that we examined earlier in this book offer us a road map for living a better, more enlightened life, but also an opportunity to make the world a more pleasant place for everyone and ensure that social justice is at its core. More and more of us are understanding and embracing how crucial it is to integrate the roots of yoga into our teaching.

There are different forms of yoga that embrace this ethos: body positive yoga, accessible yoga, yoga for all, community yoga and trauma-informed yoga, to name just a few. They may have different titles, but they share a common goal to welcome everyone to yoga and create accessibility. Body positive yoga is in alignment with many of the original teachings of yoga; for instance, it shares yoga in order to liberate the individual, which creates the unity of yoga. The paradox is that you don't have to be a yogi to practise yoga; the simplicity is that you can live a life that embodies all that it is.

Inclusive yoga communities

The future of yoga is to disrupt its current culture so that it becomes more inclusive, while the goal of yoga is to allow it to reflect the communities around us. Commercial studios have come to realise that there's a greater need for inclusivity. Although in some cases this is a result of them being called out, many have a genuine desire to be inclusive and not just fulfil a tick-box exercise. I am pleased to see that more body positive yoga classes are appearing on mainstream yoga studio timetables. More people are finally feeling welcome in the yoga space for the first time, and I really believe that this will continue.

As teachers you have a voice that is able to create yoga's future. We can all use our privilege to rebalance power dynamics so that we can start to see change. This is already starting to happen. Body positive yoga trainings and workshops are also proving popular. Alongside the amplification of voices from marginalised groups we are seeing more diversity in terms of body positive yoga teachers, which I am really pleased about.

Body positive yoga will help ensure that the teachings of yoga are shared with communities not always found in the traditional yoga space. Allies can help by sharing resources, which will enable teachers to offer mentorships and scholarships so that these skills are transferred to the communities that require them. Collective collaboration means that everyone benefits as we innovate, ensuring that no one is left behind or excluded from yoga.

All bodies in one space

The body positive movement and all those involved in making yoga more accessible are actively working to ensure that yoga is not being diluted. Yoga evolution will need creativity and innovation, which will stop the current trend of paring it back to just the asana. As my friend Jivana Heyman says, 'Accessible is the new advanced.' This eloquently describes the future of yoga; being advanced is not about getting your legs behind your head, and although asana is an important aspect of yoga it's not its whole soul.

The ability to allow every body to practise simultaneously in one space (i.e. mixed-ability classes) is the future of yoga. However, in the immediate future we will see more women-only classes or classes for Black women, as well as for other marginalised groups. This demonstrates how quickly things are changing already; a few years ago, this would have been an issue, but it's now less controversial – although still attracts negative conversations. Again, this goes back to yoga's roots. It wasn't meant to be exclusive, and its evolution means that things are returning to its original purpose of unity for all.

Body positive yoga, I hope, will soon become the norm and will no longer have to be a separate entity in order to encourage those who are invisible in the yoga space to try the practice. My wish is for online and physical yoga spaces to be rich with diversity as everyone comes together. The concept of body positivity is not a trend; it provides an actionable game plan to help change a massive societal problem.

Through body positive yoga, more and more individuals will learn the true essence of yoga. We will continue to see that yoga does not discriminate and accepts you as you are. There is absolutely nothing that you need. Just yourself: no fancy mat, no fancy clothes, just your body the way that it is.

The future is bright; the future is yoga

Body positive yoga in the UK was virtually unknown in 2015 when I started Curvesomeyoga. Now there is so much training available to equip teachers to offer accessible yoga classes to all. My dream for the future of yoga is that any student who wishes to access it can enter a classroom and have an affirming experience. Each studio or yoga space would understand how to break down barriers to wellness for marginalised people. The physical space would be accessible and welcoming; the teachers would have experience and information about how to teach to people of all shapes, sizes, ethnicities, ages and abilities in a trauma-informed and compassionate way. And every student would feel part of a community, where the practices that have been so powerful for many of us could be enjoyed by all.

Yoga has made me more flexible in mind and body, and stronger mentally and physically. I see that body positive yoga, just like the body positive movement, is a political tool for change. It's not going anywhere soon, and will be part of the future, as it becomes part of history and disrupts the yoga status quo. My hope is that one day the ethos of body positive yoga will be embraced by all styles of yoga by default, and it will be the norm for teachers to be confident in teaching students of all body types.

Diversity and inclusion will be at the heart of yoga, and I will no longer be the only person of colour in spaces where all bodies are normalised – I will see more people who look like me, as well as all ages, sizes and abilities in the spaces that I practise. My hope is that yoga will become less influenced by white supremacy and less commercialised. Instead, the focus will be less on the asana and more on yoga's rich teachings. The more these are shared, the better we will be able to ensure that social justice takes place within the world.

When this happens, we can all have a genuinely inclusive yoga world, where the underpinning teachings of yoga – the eight limbs – are part of its future and its continual evolution. I hope that yoga comes back to its true essence and that its meaning is not obscured in any way, but is understood by the many and not merely the few. Its origins will be honoured and shared authentically.

We have an opportunity to help evolve yoga in a way that eliminates any elements that are not about creating community and union. The COVID-19 pandemic has brought about so many changes to the industry – let's rebuild it on strong foundations that honour is origins together.

13

Case Studies

The following case studies are experiences shared by yoga teachers and students who are not represented in mainstream yoga. In each scenario you might want to reflect upon how you could have made these yogis feel more welcome.

AFFY UFFORT

Initially I never thought yoga was for me, and I never participated in any form of yoga. I always thought I had to be a certain shape, or size, and look a certain way before beginning any yoga practice.

My first yoga experience was in 2005. I saw a documentary on TV about hot yoga and I immediately Googled studios near me. I was so excited and signed up the very next day. I was stiff, rigid, and couldn't move anything, but the teacher was so pleasant and helpful. I slept so well that night, and I've never looked back since.

What I love about yoga is the process of connecting with your body. The time you give back to yourself to be there in the moment. The power that comes with being able to still your mind, void of unnecessary thoughts. The release, and freedom of movement, the ability to flow. What I love about yoga is endless. When I was going through some challenging periods in my life, my yoga practice helped me through them.

Most teachers were very patient, and very helpful, helping me through the postures, and correcting me, especially with the alignment. Some were a bit impatient and thought I couldn't possibly move my body. Some students would comment that I was quite good for a fat yogi! Sometimes I would correct them just to startle them, saying I wasn't fat, but strong and curvy!

I had a photoshoot and the pictures were so amazing. I was absolutely proud of myself. However, another yoga practitioner/teacher made a comment to insinuate I was overeating because my body was not typical of what yoga was about. In her words, 'And yoga is not overeating or being overweight. I really like this way of encouraging people to practise, but this is not what yoga is.'

She further added that my picture would inspire those who are overweight, which is something good, but that if I was really practising it would be impossible for me to stay as overweight, as yoga requires you to gain control over all your addictions, including eating habits. So literally without knowing me she had come to the conclusion that I was overweight, I had an addiction, and I wasn't practising yoga because I wasn't as skinny as she was. It was a bit disappointing to witness such unintelligent thoughts and words.

Yes, teachers and students make assumptions based on my body. I get 'looks'. I was once at the front row of a class and the teacher asked me to move to the back because she thought I was new, and she wanted the people in the front to help lead the class. I told her no. At the end of the class she came up to me and said I had an amazing yoga practice for a 'person my size'. She just flat-out spoilt the compliment.

TARA TOMES

I've always loved the idea of yoga: spending an hour on the mat and forgetting about the stresses of daily life. Despite only ever seeing skinny women who look great in leggings and a crop top doing yoga, I didn't let those stereotypes put me off trying it. I think that any kind of fitness should be open to everyone.

I'd tried yoga a few times over the years and didn't really feel like I needed anything before attending classes. In actual fact, one thing that would have really helped me enjoy them more was learning the poses and modifications so that I didn't have to rely on teachers to spot that I was struggling. I find that teachers assume that breaking it down makes it easy, but that isn't always the case; often, understanding the 'end goal' makes it much easier to work out how to get your body there and if, in fact, you can't, how to find an alternative way.

It wasn't until I found Curvesomeyoga that I felt a teacher really understood the challenges faced by someone who's bigger; learning those modified poses, as well as how to use props, was a game-changer.

To be honest, before I found Curvesomeyoga I hadn't even considered that yoga classes needed to be more inclusive or accessible. I just assumed that because I was plus size I would always struggle, but that's absolutely not the case. The classes I'd attended were great, don't get me wrong, but they could have done so much more to welcome people of all body types, shapes and levels of ability. I never even knew that things like chair and bed yoga existed, and I think they would just be so life-changing for someone with limited mobility.

In the classes themselves, the teachers went at quite a speed and were so focused on the flow that they didn't look around to identify who might need additional support or suggestions. No one wants to feel like the failing kid in the class, but simply acknowledging there are other ways to achieve the same benefits as the 'standard' pose really does make all the difference.

My first experience of yoga was when I was at university; I joined the campus gym and gave a few different classes a go. I liked the essence of it, but I always wanted to try yoga as I'd seen so many people talk about how much they loved it. It wasn't until a few years later that I went to a yoga class, but I walked out really disappointed that it hadn't lived up to expectations. The class was far too quick, despite being billed a beginner's class, and I didn't feel any benefits whatsoever. It didn't put me off trying yoga again but it definitely could have.

Until I found Curvesomeyoga only one teacher had ever actually 'taught' me. She saw me struggling with downward dog and showed me how to do it against a wall. Really, she could have just shown me how to use the blocks, but I still applaud her for recognising my struggle and trying to help.

What I've always found is that teachers very much stand at the front of the class and lead, rather than spending time in among their yogis helping them to truly reap the benefits of yoga. They might dip in every now and then to move someone's leg into position, but I never found that they were there to take us all on a journey.

Donna changed all of that – every class is like being told a story: learning the true benefits of yoga, why the stereotypes aren't a true representation of its origins and, most importantly, how to take yoga into your daily life.

My main experience with yoga was just an expectation that everyone in the room would be able to do the same move and if you couldn't, you probably weren't flexible enough. It's a sad feeling being at the back of the class feeling hot and frustrated that you can't do it and no one explaining that, even in a bigger body, yoga is absolutely for you and that you can find your own flow.

I committed to weekly yoga at a local studio because a colleague and I used to go together before work. It was run by a really lovely girl who was so passionate about it, which made it a wonderful experience, and the studio only held 12 people so it was always a nice intimate environment.

However, finding Curvesomeyoga was a real game-changer! I'd come home from another class feeling frustrated that yoga wasn't living up to my expectations and I was almost ready to give up on it altogether. I decided to Google 'plus size yoga' and stumbled across the Curvesomeyoga YouTube video. It was the first time I'd seen someone over a size 14 doing yoga, as well as the first time I'd seen that there were modifications. I suddenly felt there was hope so I went onto Curvesomeyoga's Instagram and saw the 30x30 challenge [a yoga challenge that consisted of 30 minutes x 30 days of yoga]. I decided to dive in and sign up!

People make assumptions about my body – I saw this even more when I started sharing my yoga journey on my own Instagram account; people were so supportive and complimentary but, actually, I think they were mostly shocked that a big girl could actually *do* yoga and look good doing it.

If you're a bigger girl, or maybe someone who isn't able bodied, and you don't have the confidence, I just don't think you'll stick at yoga unless you find a supportive community and teacher like Curvesomeyoga and Donna.

The yoga industry is not as diverse as it could be, but I'm certainly seeing a wider range of yogis on Instagram, which is really encouraging. It's a case of finding your people and seeking out yoga teachers and classes that work for you. There's a lot of work to do in the media and with fitness brands – even those who do plus sizes – but we're getting there with baby steps.

My advice for anyone looking to start yoga is just give it a go! Leave the preconceptions and stereotypes behind – get on the mat, do research beforehand if that helps you, and just move your body. Yoga is an incredibly powerful community so find your people and find your flow.

Nothing prevented me from starting yoga, but I'm a pretty confident person, so I've never minded being the worst in the class. I think the idea of yoga and being someone who loved it always outshone the hesitation around whether it was for me or not.

ELAINE HUGHES

Unfortunately I did not believe that yoga was for me. I had tried going to classes in the past, but have always felt out of place. Before starting my yoga journey I feel that I needed to learn more about the process and try to find accessible locations, or empathetic teachers.

The yoga classes that I have attended have not been inclusive. I haven't found any inclusive body positive yoga classes or teachers.

My first yoga class was in Coventry, and I found that I was judged from the moment I walked in, when I explained that I couldn't do certain poses due to my physical disability. I was constantly berated and told that yoga wasn't suitable for me as I needed to complete the postures to get any benefit at all. Some teachers refused to interact with me as they felt I would not be able to do the poses at the same level as the other students.

The stereotypes I encountered resulted because I was in a primarily white town and as a Black disabled woman I felt very uncomfortable and judged both for my limitations and as the only Black woman in the class. I have been told classes are inclusive but in reality they were not and as a result have experienced microaggressions.

I haven't been back to a studio since my last encounter, but when I have mentioned that I have done armchair yoga at home by watching YouTube, I have had comments that this isn't correct yoga and it's not actually doing my body any good in the long run. I have been told I need to be in a proper yoga class to achieve the full benefits. I have since learnt that it's actually very inclusive for people with all levels of ability, and there are people like Donna who are inclusive and breaking down the myths around it. This is what I love about yoga.

The stereotype the yoga industry projects is not diverse, but I am learning and seeing more yoga teachers like Donna who show how inclusive it can be and encourage diversity.

For anyone wishing to try yoga I would say do your research

and really have a conversation with your class tutor or other friends/family to help you locate one. Once you're comfortable with this it will make it easier. I had been prevented from starting yoga because of a lack of confidence and not finding accessible locations and tutors with a diverse audience.

JUNIOR VALENTINE

I felt yoga was for me; it was something I wanted to try nine-plus years ago so I went searching, but it seemed yoga classes weren't easy to find. I felt that I wanted to improve flexibility and strength but when I really delved deeper I found that yoga was so much more than that; but the idea of yoga was probably at the forefront of my mind, like a meditating yogi.

Generally speaking the classes I attend are not body positive, because the people who are teaching are teaching from their experience really – if they don't have your body type they don't necessarily understand your challenge, but there are options and modifications in some classes I attend.

I actually hated yoga back in 2008. We had to do it as a part of my performing arts degree, but I just wanted to do our regular dance class. It was taught by our dance teacher, but I feel I was not in the right space. It was really a case of being new and at the beginning of something thinking I was failing at it. But I'm glad I continued.

Yoga for me is a feeling sensation; the magic is in the moments of stillness, or self-realisation in a class. The true essence of yoga that can be discovered is something I also love, and how its simple teachings can apply in so many ways.

I'm a reader of energy; I had to go to a class to get a feeling for whether the teacher was for me. Generally I've had good experiences, but I'm a quick detector of nonsense so I won't stick around or even attend if the class doesn't feel right. For instance, I'm not a fan of Triyoga so I don't attend classes at their studio. It's definitely not my vibe or tribe.

Unfortunately I feel these stereotypes and microaggressions are and will always be there. People have assumed that I'm a beginner when I come into class, but when I explain I am a teacher they change their attitude.

I believe we all make assumptions, because of preconceived notions and all this programming which we have to unlearn because it's harmful. Just because someone has a bigger body, a lot of people assume they aren't flexible, and same on the other side – it should not be assumed that if they are too thin they naturally have muscle strength. A good example is the dance world: everyone always asks a dancer if they can do the splits, as if that will authenticate them as a dancer, but all of our bodies vary and what they can do varies. Folks have to check their biases at the door and go off what's in front of them in the present.

Personally, I look for a teacher who is honest in what they teach; as a teacher I can't stand all this love and light BS so I talk about the challenges and the shadow, because sometimes that's where a lot of us are. So if someone is too in the air energy I tend not to be around them or go to that type of teacher's class.

Worldwide, hell no, the yoga world is not diverse – ask any yogis to name famous teachers and they are normally always white. There is just about only Jonelle or Dianne that folks can name as Black teachers. What about famous South Asian teachers? I would bet yoga folks couldn't even name one.

It's too Westernised as a money-making machine, and it's white centred because they have seen a business money-making model and have continued to perpetuate it, but I know you and others are working hard to rewire the way it's been and I applaud that.

I would recommend anyone wanting to do yoga to try as many intro deals and studios as you can until you find your style and teacher. Go to the teacher's class you can't pronounce, or the teacher who doesn't look like a typical Suzy, try various styles so that you can get a full experience of yoga, and there are so many.

In 2008 yoga was around, but wasn't as accessible as it is now. With it now being so accessible I hope the studios are sending out the message that yoga is for everyone.

SASKIA BOLSCHER

I have always felt that yoga was for me. Sometimes I tend to go to any class I feel drawn to; however, after the lockdown weight gain I'm finding it harder to keep up with the typical Vinyasa class. Yoga makes me feel calm, balanced, in the moment.

I look for teachers who hold space for any and all students, and who don't rush through a class, so there is enough time for everyone to get into poses. Ideally also someone who offers different options for different poses, so that everyone can join in.

The yoga industry is starting to look more diverse, but at the core it's still very much mainly thin, white, young, flexible women. This is why my classes are targeted towards curvier people – I want people to see that yoga is for anyone.

Contributors

Saskia Bolscher is a body positive, curvy yoga teacher who is passionate about making yoga inclusive and accessible for everybody. She teaches Hatha, yin and slow flows.

> Website: yogawithsaskia.co.uk
> Instagram: www.instagram.com/yogawithsaskia

Armani Eke has had a yoga practice spanning 13 years and has been teaching adults, children and teens for the last seven years. In addition to her yoga certifications, she has trained to teach mindfulness, meditation and breathwork. She focuses on bringing wellness practices to under-served and under-represented communities.

Elaine Hughes is an entrepreneur and professional speaker. Born with spastic quadriplegic cerebral palsy, her mobility and ability to co-ordinate physically are seriously compromised, alongside chronic pain.

Elaine advocates for the disabled community on a variety of issues including housing, employment, disability rights, and so on. She is passionate about supporting young carers within Black communities who don't have a voice.

Elaine is a professional speaker who has appeared on numerous panels talking about her experiences as a disabled entrepreneur. She is a Disability Champion, advocating for disabled entrepreneurs to start ecommerce businesses and advising organisations to support disabled employees in the workplace.

Subramaniam Manoharan (aka Mano) is a 71-year-old yoga teacher who discovered yoga the age of 46 while working as an electronic system engineer.

Mano did a beginners yoga course at the Sivananda Centre in Putney. In 1997 he completed his teacher training course at the Sivananda Ashram in Kerala, and in 2001 completed the advanced teacher training. Mano's passion for yoga has meant that he has been teaching yoga since 1997.

Heather Mason is the founder of The Minded Institute, a leading yoga therapy training school in the UK, and the Yoga in Healthcare Alliance. Committed to bringing yoga into health systems, she has also taught in medical schools, educating future doctors in integrating yoga into treatment, and continues to lecture at various universities on this topic. Heather is the secretariat for the All Party Parliamentary Group on Yoga in Society in the UK. She is an RYT-500 and C-Physiology, and has done extensive study in neuroscience.

Website: www.themindedinstitute.com

Aisha Nash left a career working in Michelin-starred restaurants after the stress of the job caught up with both her body and her mind. She discovered yoga and wanted to share the practice that helped her be entirely content with exactly the person she is, but found that she didn't feel like she fitted the mould of a yoga teacher that studios were looking for. Aisha now teaches classes that are focused on inclusivity, diversity and self-love, with what she calls her Anti-Diet Yoga approach.

Gabi Parkham (she/her) is a yoga teacher who has been practising yoga since childhood and teaching for over seven years. She is passionate about finding equity and justice through yoga and making yoga accessible to as many people as possible. Since coming out as bisexual at the age of 18, Gabi has been an active LGBTQIA equity educator and consultant, leading LGBTQIA trainings in schools, youth movements, for perinatal professionals, and for civil servants.

In 2018 Gabi co-founded Laviot (www.laviot.org), a social and supportive community for LGBTQIA Jewish women and non-binary people. Gabi believes that yoga classes and studios should be spaces free from assumptions, microaggressions and discrimination, so she regularly runs workshops for movement teachers and studios who want to make their spaces more welcoming for the LGBTQIA community.

Ava Riby-Williams is a queer, Ghanaian and Indian artist, community facilitator, activist, yoga teacher and student, living in London. Her work focuses on using creativity to connect, and guiding groups into deeper contemplation about issues concerning their liberation and wellbeing, on personal and collective levels. As a guide, Ava is clear that the point of her work is to encourage students to become their own inner teachers: she does this with young people and adults.

Ava is driven by the importance of making healing practices accessible to isolated and marginalised communities as a tool to unwind trauma; she has been facilitating and creating trainings in this field since 2017.

With over ten years of yoga, creative practice, facilitation and performance experience, her teaching is often woven with song, poetry and play as a way to deepen our capacity to love and experience life.

Tara Tomes is a PR expert and entrepreneur based in Birmingham who is passionate about people, purpose and paying-it-forward. She founded the award-winning EAST VILLAGE. back in 2013, as an agency centred around team culture, putting flexible working, free mental health support, and DEI (diversity, equity and inclusion) at the top of the priority list.

In addition to running the agency, Tara provides one-to-one consultancy to founders of businesses, helping them to power up their personal brand and step into the media spotlight. She is an advocate for making the PR industry more diverse and is a founding member of BPFS Black Leaders Network, a collective of established leaders who share expertise and best practice to help businesses change their approach to DEI.

Passionate about giving time to things that matter, Tara is a non-executive director at TAG Network West Midlands, as well as co-founder and trustee of the homeless charity Let's Feed Brum. She sits on the management committee for Tabor Living, a homeless accommodation provider, and is patron for the drop-in centre SIFA Fireside.

Affy Uffort is a health and wellness entrepreneur who runs several successful businesses under her company AffyBaLE Group. She is an avid yoga enthusiast who has been practising for over 16 years. Her passion is to help people lead a happy and peaceful existence.

Junior Valentine is a proud South London native born and bred with a background in performing. His mission is to connect with as many souls as he can, and he offers healing and support through various mediums, whether that be sound, yoga, massage or energy healing work.

Responsibility for healing lands in our own laps, and working through these mediums helps to bring forth change, growth and the breaking of cycles. It doesn't mean it will be easy! But Junior knows deep down it's worth it, and he believes knowledge of how to do this should be shared with everyone.

Website: www.juniorvalentine.co.uk

Author contact

https://thenobleartofyoga.co.uk
Instagram and Facebook: @donnanobleyoga and @curvesomeyoga
Email: me@donnanobleyoga.co.uk

References and Resources

ANLP International CIC (n.d.) 'Definition of NLP'. https://anlp.org/knowledge-base/definition-of-nlp (retrieved on 23 November 2021).

Ashby, M. (2006) *The African Origins of Hatha Yoga.* Miami, FL: Cruzian Mystic Books/Sema Institute of Yoga.

Association for Size Diversity and Health (ASDAH) (2020) 'The Health at Every Size® (HAES®) Approach'. https://asdah.org/health-at-every-size-haes-approach (retrieved on 7 December 2021).

Barkataki, S. (2020) *Embrace Yoga's Roots: Courageous Ways to Deepen Your Yoga Practice.* Orlando, FL: Ignite Yoga and Wellness Institute.

Bell, C. (2018, 8 March) 'Women in Yoga: A Short History'. Hugger Mugger [Blog]. www.huggermugger.com/blog/2018/women-in-yoga-short-history (retrieved on 23 November 2021).

Branch, T. (1968) 'Citizen King Transcript'. *PBS.* Archived from the original on 25 January 2013. https://web.archive.org/web/20130125144003/http://www.pbs.org/wgbh/amex/mlk/filmmore/pt.html (retrieved on 23 November 2021).

Brumfitt, T. (dir.) (2016) *Embrace* [Film]. Transmission Films.

Cherry, K. (2020, 13 December) 'What Is Othering?' Verywell Mind. www.verywellmind.com/what-is-othering-5084425 (retrieved on 5 December 2021).

Coughlin, D. (2014, 11 October) 'Fat girls do yoga too'. *Guardian*, 11 October. www.theguardian.com/lifeandstyle/2014/oct/11/fat-girls-do-yoga-too (retrieved on 23 November 2021).

Crawford, R. (1980) 'Healthism and the medicalization of everyday life'. *International Journal of Health Services 10*(3): 365–388.

Feuerstein, G. (1998) *The Yoga Tradition: Its History, Literature, Philosophy and Practice.* Prescott, AZ: Hohm Press.

Fossella, T. and Welwood, J. (2011) *Human Nature, Buddha Nature: An Interview with John Welwood.* www.johnwelwood.com/articles/TRIC_interview_uncut.pdf (retrieved on 23 November 2021).

Heyman, J. (2019) *Accessible Yoga.* Boulder, CO: Shambhala.

Johnson, M. C. (2020) *Skill in Action: Radicalizing Your Yoga Practice to Create a Just World.* Boulder, CO: Shambhala.

Kemetic YogaSkills (n.d.) 'History of Kemetic Yoga.' https://kemeticyogaskills.com/history-of-kemetic-yoga (retrieved on 23 November 2021).

Lau, A. (2021, 11 January) 'The rise of fad diets'. *CNBC.* www.cnbc.com/video/2021/01/11/how-dieting-became-a-71-billion-industry-from-atkins-and-paleo-to-noom.html (retrieved on 23 November 2021).

Loeber, S., Burgmer, R., Wyssen, A., Leins, J. *et al.* (2016) 'Short-term effects of media exposure to the thin ideal in female inpatients with an eating disorder compared to female inpatients with a mood or anxiety disorder or women with no psychiatric disorder'. *International Journal of Eating Disorders 49*(7): 708–715.

National Institute of Neurological Disorders and Stroke (2019) 'Bell's Palsy Information Page'. www.ninds.nih.gov/Disorders/All-Disorders/Bells-Palsy-Information-Page (retrieved on 9 December 2021).

NCCIH (National Center for Complementary and Integrative Health) (2021) 'Yoga: What You Need to Know'. www.nccih.nih.gov/health/yoga-what-you-need-to-know (retrieved on 23 November 2021).

Office of Diversity and Outreach (n.d.) 'What Is Unconscious Bias?' https://diversity.ucsf.edu/resources/unconscious-bias (retrieved on 23 November 2021).

Parker, G. (2020) *Restorative Yoga for Ethnic and Race-Based Stress and Trauma.* London: Singing Dragon.

Powell, S. (2018, 16 June) 'The ancient yoga strap'. The Luminescent. www.theluminescent.org/2018/06/the-ancient-yoga-strap-yogapatta.html

Remski, M. (2019a) *Practice and All Is Coming: Abuse, Cult Dynamics, and Healing in Yoga and Beyond.* Rangiora, New Zealand: Embodied Wisdom Publishing.

Remski, M. (2019b) '*On "Practice and All is Coming": Matthew Remski interviewed by Donna Noble.*' http://matthewremski.com/wordpress/on-practice-and-all-is-coming-matthew-remski-interviewed-by-donna-noble (retrieved on 18 January 2022).

Somé, S. (2000) *The Spirit of Intimacy: Ancient Teachings in the Ways of Relationships.* New York, NY: William Morrow & Company.

Streeter, C. C., Gerbarg, P. L., Saper, R. B., Ciraulo, D. A. and Brown, R. P. (2012) 'Effects of yoga on the autonomic nervous system, gamma-aminobutyric-acid, and allostasis in epilepsy, depression, and post-traumatic stress disorder.' *Medical Hypotheses 78*(5): 571–579.

World Health Organization (2018) 'Mental health: Strengthening our response'. www.who.int/news-room/fact-sheets/detail/mental-health-strengthening-our-response (retrieved on 19 January 2022).

Yoga and Body Image Coalition (2014, 1 December) 'This Is What a Yogi Looks Like'. http://ybicoalition.com/this-is-what-a-yogi-looks-like (retrieved on 23 November 2021).

Recommended books

Bondy, D. (2019) *Yoga for Everyone: 50 Poses for Every Type of Body*. Indianapolis, IN: DK Publishing.

Bondy, D. and Heagberg, K. (2020) *Yoga Where You Are*. Boulder, CO: Shambhala.

Heyman, J. (2019) *Accessible Yoga*. Boulder, CO: Shambhala.

Martin, M. (2019) *Can Everyone Please Calm Down?: A Guide to 21st Century Sexuality*. London: Hachette Children's Group.

Read, N. (2021) *The Good Ally*. London: HarperCollins.

Saad, L. F. (2020) *Me and White Supremacy*. London: Quercus Books.

Strings, S. (2019) *Fearing the Black Body: The Racial Origins of Fat Phobia*. New York, NY: New York University Press.

Resources
Curvesomeyoga Plus Size Yoga introduction video

https://youtu.be/XFxfuOo_BkU

Eat Breathe Thrive

A not-for-profit organisation that offers courses on yoga and eating disorders.

www.eatbreathethrive.org

Off the Mat Into the World

A community of leaders bridging yoga and activism, who train on subjects such as trauma, social justice, cultural appropriation and body image.

www.offthematintotheworld.org

Stonewall

An organisation dedicated to supporting LGBTQIA people.

www.stonewall.org.uk

The Minded Institute

Provides yoga therapy education to yoga and health professionals.

https://themindedinstitute.com

Trans Yoga Project

A collaborative that supports trans people's spiritual wellness through education, advocacy and community building.

https://transyogaproject.com

Yoga for Humankind

A training organisation and global community dedicated to trauma-informed education and change.

https://yogaforhumankind.org

Yogamatters
Retailer of yoga and wellbeing items.

www.yogamatters.com

Index